KU-033-647

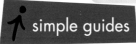

simple guides

Irritable bowel syndrome

Dr Eleanor Bull

Dr Richard Stevens

Irritable bowel syndrome
First published – April 2006

Published by
CSF Medical Communications Ltd
1 Bankside, Lodge Road, Long Hanborough
Oxfordshire, OX29 8LJ, UK
T +44 (0)1993 885370 F +44 (0)1993 881868
enquiries@bestmedicine.com
www.bestmedicine.com

We are always interested in hearing from anyone
who has anything to add to our Simple Guides.
Please send your comments to *editor@csfmedical.com*.

Author Dr Eleanor Bull
Managing Editor Dr Eleanor Bull
Medical Editor Dr Richard Stevens
Science Editor Dr Scott Chambers
Production Editor Emma Catherall
Layout Jamie McCansh and Julie Smith
Operations Manager Julia Savory
Publisher Stephen I'Anson

ISBN-10: 1-905466-08-0
ISBN-13: 978-190546-608-5

Printed in Italy.

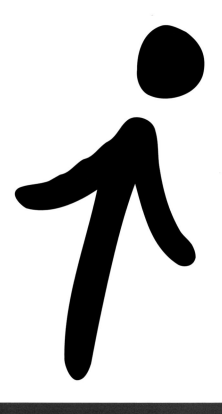

FOREWORD

TRISHA MACNAIR

Doctor and BBC Health Journalist

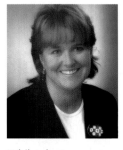 Getting involved in managing your own medical condition – or helping those you love or care for to manage theirs – is a vital step towards keeping as healthy as possible. Whilst doctors, nurses and the rest of your healthcare team can help you with expert advice and guidance, nobody knows your body, your symptoms and what is right for *you* as well as you do.

There is no long-term (chronic) medical condition or illness that I can think of where the person concerned has absolutely no influence at all on their situation. The way you choose to live your life, from the food you eat to the exercise you take, will impact upon your disease, your well-being and how able you are to cope. You are in charge!

Being involved in making choices about your treatment helps you to feel in control of your problems, and makes sure you get the help that you really need. Research clearly shows that when people living with a chronic illness take an active role in looking after themselves, they can bring about significant improvements in their illness and vastly improve the quality of life they enjoy.

Of course, there may be occasions when you feel particularly unwell and it all seems out of your control. Yet most of the time there are plenty of things that you can do in order to reduce the negative effects that your condition can have on your life. This way you feel as good as possible and may even be able to alter the course of your condition.

So how do you gain the confidence and skills to take an active part in managing your condition, communicate with health professionals and work through sometimes worrying and emotive issues? The answer is to become better informed. Reading about your problem, talking to others who have been through similar experiences and hearing what the experts have to say will all help to build up your understanding and help you to take an active role in your own health care.

Simple Guides provide an invaluable source of help, giving you the facts that you need in order to understand the key issues and discuss them with your doctors and other professionals involved in your care. The information is presented in an accessible way but without neglecting the important details. Produced independently and under the guidance of medical experts *Irritable bowel syndrome* is an evidence-based, balanced and up-to-date review that I hope you will find enables you to play an active part in the successful management of your condition.

What happens normally?

WHAT HAPPENS NORMALLY?

The food we eat is not in a form that the body can use for nourishment. Digestion is the process by which food is broken down into its smallest parts so that the body can use it to release energy.

WHY DO WE NEED TO EAT?

We use energy in everything we do, right down to turning the pages of this book. Food is our main source of energy. This is because the chemical bonds that link food molecules together store energy. When the bonds are broken – when we eat and digest food – energy is released.

The energy value of food is expressed in calories. Different foods release different amounts of energy when they are digested.

- Carbohydrates (found in bread, potatoes, rice, pasta, fruits and vegetables) have about four calories per gram.

- Proteins (found in meat, eggs and beans) have about four calories per gram.

- Fat (found in meats, butter, milk and cheese) contains about twice as many calories per gram as protein or carbohydrate. Fat molecules are therefore a rich source of energy for the body.

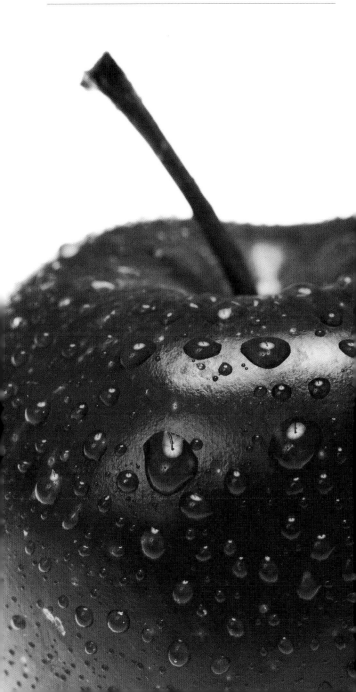

THE DIGESTIVE TRACT AND THE PROCESS OF DIGESTION

The digestive tract is the part of the body that processes food. Put simply, it is a hollow tube that runs between the mouth and the anus. The actual length of the tract is a startling 5 metres, so you can imagine the extent to which it must be twisted and coiled inside the body.

Digestion describes the conversion of food into a form that can be easily absorbed by the body. In a nutshell, food enters through the mouth and waste products are removed from the body through the anus after digestion has taken place. The process can be described in ten basic stages.

1. Food is chewed and partly broken down by the teeth.

2. Saliva in the mouth helps to kick-start the digestive process.

3. The partially digested food is swallowed. At this point we stop controlling the digestive process ourselves and our body takes over.

4. The food mixture is forced down the oesophagus towards the stomach by a process called **peristalsis**.

5. In the stomach, a watery fluid called gastric juice mixes with the food to form chyme – a puréed mixture.

6. The stomach works like a gate and a mixer by gradually churning and releasing food into the small intestine at a rate that is slow enough to make sure that it is properly digested.

7. The small intestine extends up to 3 metres in length but is tightly coiled in the body. It is here where most of the digestion occurs. Useful substances like water, vitamins and minerals are absorbed from the small intestine into the body via the bloodstream. To help it to digest food, the small intestine uses substances made by the pancreas and liver, called pancreatic juice and bile.

8. The small intestine gives way to the large intestine, sometimes known as the colon. The large intestine is wider than the small intestine, but is shorter, measuring about 1.5 metres. No digestion takes place here but water that has been squeezed out of food is absorbed into the body.

9. The remaining undigested food, now a waste product, is propelled by peristalsis to the rectum where it is stored.

10. When the rectum is stretched sufficiently, it prompts a bowel movement and the waste leaves the body as faeces.

PERISTALSIS

Peristalsis (*per-ih-stawl-sis*) describes the 'rippling' movements that push food and liquid through the digestive tract. The walls of the digestive tract contain muscle. During digestion, a bit like squeezing toothpaste out of a tube, the muscles behind and in front of the food parcel alternately contract and then relax to force it onwards towards the stomach. Peristalsis is an involuntary process – once we have swallowed the food, the body takes over – and we are unaware that it is taking place.

Unlike us, cows and other cud-chewing animals are able to reverse the direction of peristalsis when necessary, bringing food up from the stomach to the mouth for a few extra chomps to speed up digestion.

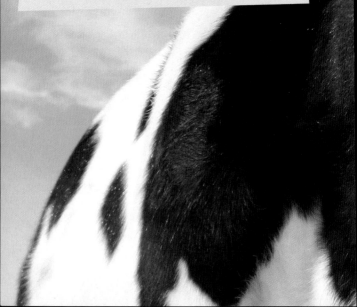

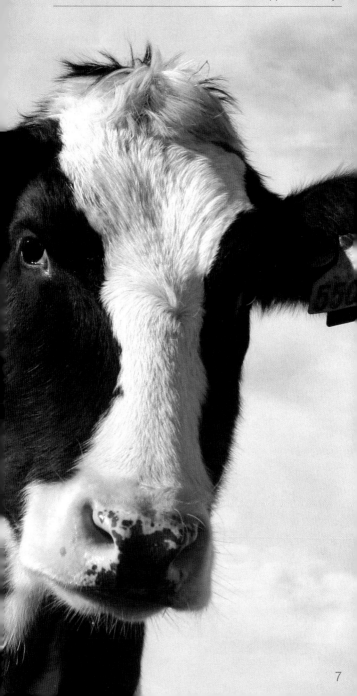

THE BOTTOM LINE

The bowel (made up of the small and large intestines) is the long tube that runs from your stomach to your back passage (rectum). They function to firstly break down and digest food so nutrients can pass into your bloodstream (small intestine) and then to carry away the waste products (large intestine).

It usually takes up to 48 hours for the contents of the large intestine to travel down to the rectum. But if the waste products travel too slowly, too much water is reabsorbed into the body and they become hard and dry. This can lead to constipation. Conversely, if waste moves through the large intestine too quickly then not enough water is absorbed and diarrhoea results.

Although it can be noisy and embarrassing, passing wind is an inevitable (and important) part of digestion. It is the body's way of getting rid of any air that we have inadvertently swallowed whilst eating and also the gas that is produced during digestion. Passing wind helps to lower the pressure within the digestive tract and prevents painful stretching of the intestines. As we are all aware, some foods (like beans, cabbage and broccoli) are more likely to produce wind than others and this is because they increase the amount of intestinal gas produced during digestion.

Although we may not like to admit it, we pass wind about 15 to 25 times a day.

TERMINOLOGY

Abdomen	The tummy or belly.
Anus	The back passage; lower opening of the gut.
Bowels	The small and large intestines, collectively.
Colon	The large intestine.
Colonic	Relating to the large intestine.
Duodenum	The part of the small intestine leading from the stomach.
Gastric	Having to do with the stomach.
Gastrointestinal	Having to do with the digestive tract.
Gastrointestinal tract	The part of the digestive system that includes the mouth, oesophagus, stomach and intestines.
Gut	Intestines.
Ileum	The lower half of the small intestine.
Jejunum	The upper half of small intestine between the duodenum and the ileum. Most food is absorbed here.
Large intestine	The part of the digestive tract leading from the ileum of the small intestine to the anus. Also known as the colon.
Small intestine	The part of the digestive tract leading from the stomach to the large intestine. It is here that most digestion takes place.
Oesophagus	The food pipe that runs between the throat and the stomach.
Rectum	The lower end of the digestive tract leading from the colon to the anus.
Stomach	A sac-like organ between the oesophagus and the small intestine that churns and breaks down food, with the help of gastric juices.

This *Simple Guide* will explain what goes wrong with your bowels if you have irritable bowel syndrome (IBS) and give you the information you need to make sure it is managed as well as it can be.

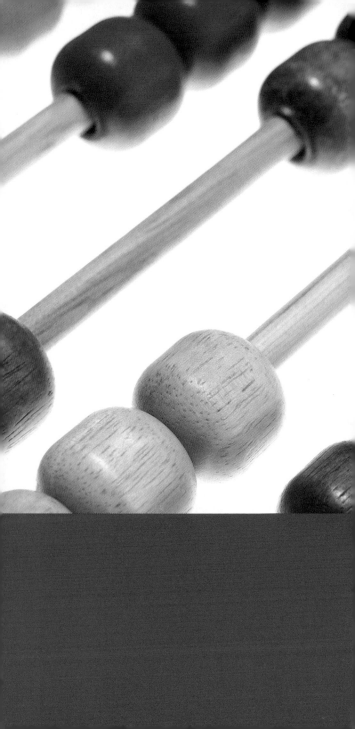

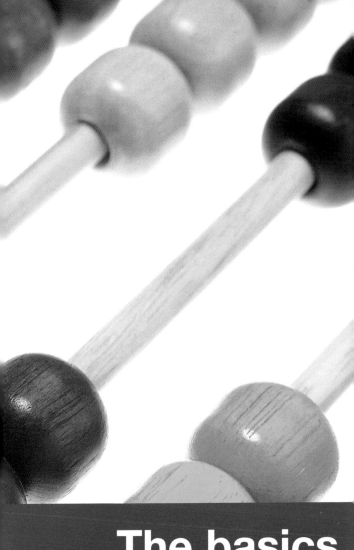

The basics

IRRITABLE BOWEL SYNDROME – THE BASICS

Nobody enjoys divulging their bathroom habits. Yet, when you suffer from a disorder like IBS it is often very difficult to conceal what's going on from friends, work colleagues or even strangers in the street.

People with irritable bowel syndrome (often shortened to IBS) suffer from recurring bouts of abdominal pain that can lead to diarrhoea, constipation or a mixture of the two. Either way, people with IBS usually end up spending a lot of time in the toilet. Although IBS is not life-threatening, it can certainly make life difficult and deal a significant blow to your self-confidence. Even relatively simple tasks, like catching the bus to work, can become virtually impossible on bad days.

People with IBS often:

■ feel very self-conscious
■ have low self-confidence
■ try to hide their condition from those around them.

IBS can stop you from:

■ going to work
■ socialising
■ eating the foods you enjoy.

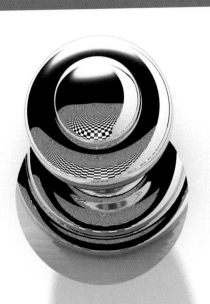

**DO
NOT
DISTURB!**

SYMPTOMS

The symptoms of IBS vary hugely from person to person, ranging from barely noticeable to completely debilitating. For women, you may have noticed that your symptoms may get worse around the time of your period. Sometimes even the weather can make things worse. Generally speaking, the 'colonic' symptoms of IBS can include:

- abdominal pain or cramping
- changes in bowel function, usually resulting in diarrhoea or constipation
- mucus in the stools
- a feeling that you may not make it to the toilet in time
- a feeling of incomplete evacuation when you do make it to the toilet
- a bloated, sticking out stomach
- wind
- embarrassing rumbling noises.

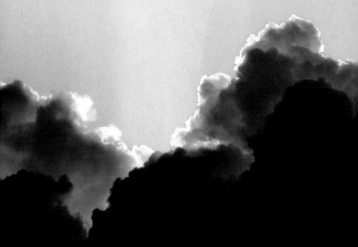

THE FOUR KEY SYMPTOMS OF IBS

Pain, constipation, diarrhoea, abdominal bloating.
The Primary Care Society for Gastroenterology

Other 'non-colonic' symptoms associated with IBS
can include:

- backache
- tiredness
- nausea and vomiting
- heartburn
- pain when having sex
- pain when urinating
- anxiety
- depression.

WHAT MAKES IBS PAINFUL?

Nearly all people with IBS will suffer from bouts of extreme pain in their abdomen. This abdominal pain or cramping is arguably the most unpleasant symptom of IBS and is the symptom which most often drives people to visit their GP. The pain is often described as either nagging and sharp, or heavy and dull. It can come on in waves and is usually worse on the left hand side of the body. Going to the toilet can often provide some form of relief but this is usually short-lived.

People with IBS are often classified according to the symptom they suffer from the most. The three main types of IBS are:

1. constipation-predominant IBS

2. diarrhoea-predominant IBS

3. mixed type IBS (alternating constipation and diarrhoea).

The type of IBS you suffer from dictates the way in which it will be treated. Although all three types are relatively common, mixed type IBS tends to affect the most people (approximately 39%) compared with constipation- (34%) and diarrhoea-predominant IBS (27%).

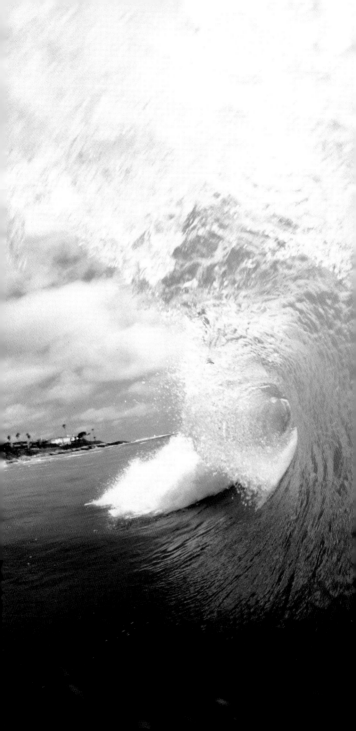

WHAT DOES HAVING IBS MEAN?

This is a difficult question to answer because IBS
affects different people in very different ways.
Some people only experience mild symptoms for
short periods (occasional 'flare ups'), whilst others
have unpleasant symptoms that persist for a long
time. Either way, it is probable that IBS will remain
with you for the rest of your life – it is a chronic
(long-term) condition.

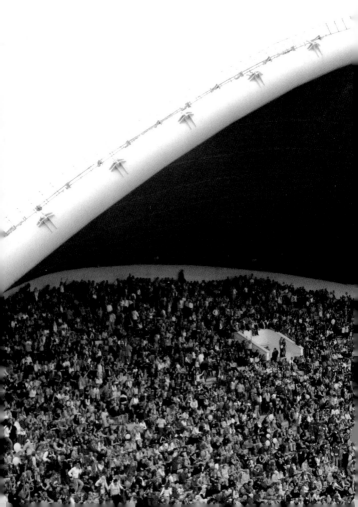

FIVE THINGS YOU MAY NOT KNOW ABOUT IBS

1. IBS affects millions of people in the UK (about 1 in 5 of us).

2. IBS is the most common gastrointestinal condition seen by GPs.

3. IBS will not develop into cancer.

4. IBS is rarely caused by an allergy to food.

5. IBS is also known as spastic colon, spastic colitis, mucous colitis, nervous diarrhoea or nervous colon (although strictly speaking, some of these names are not entirely accurate).

WHAT CAUSES IBS?

No-one is sure exactly what causes IBS. In fact, in most people IBS can be put down to any one of a number of things. For whatever reason, the gastrointestinal tract functions differently in people with IBS. Some people believe that:

■ people with IBS have an over-sensitive gastrointestinal tract

■ IBS stems from a problem with the nerves that control the bowels

■ the bowel muscles work differently in people with IBS.

Ultimately, this means that people who have IBS process food more slowly or more quickly than normal. If the bowels process waste too slowly, then it can cause constipation, whereas if the waste is processed too quickly diarrhoea can result.

WHAT TRIGGERS THE SYMPTOMS OF IBS?

A trigger is something that worsens or brings on the symptoms of IBS, but is not what causes IBS in the first place. Different people link their IBS to different things. As we will see, most IBS treatments are centred on removing these triggers or reducing their impact.

Possible IBS triggers can include:

- stress (like trouble at work or marital problems)

- certain types of food (true food allergies are rare but some people with IBS may be intolerant to foods like wheat and some dairy products)

- alcohol

- caffeine

- smoking

- a bout of gastroenteritis (known as post-infective IBS)

- certain types of medication.

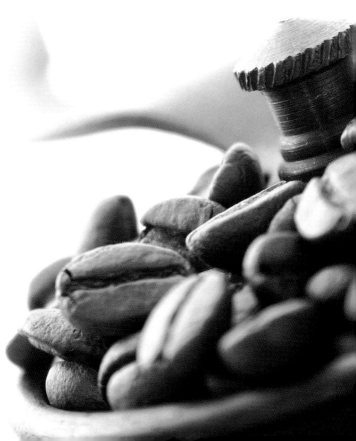

DIAGNOSING IBS

Although most people find that they are able to manage their IBS without having to visit their GP, if you feel that your symptoms are so severe that they are starting to seriously affect the way you live your life, it is important that you seek medical advice.

There is no simple test for IBS. When you see your doctor they will usually ask you about your symptoms and your medical history and they may examine your abdomen and/or back passage.

For many people, it is a relief to have someone to talk to about their symptoms and to take them seriously. Having a doctor confirm that there is a name for their condition and realising that there is help available to treat it, can make a real difference.

Sometimes, your doctor may refer you to a specialist (called a gastroenterologist) for further tests. This is usually so that they can exclude more serious bowel problems that can produce similar symptoms to IBS. However, referral is usually only necessary for:

- older people (over the age of 45 years)
- people who have abnormal symptoms (i.e. sudden weight loss, blood in the stools, symptoms that occur at night)
- people with a history of gastrointestinal (particularly colorectal) cancer in their family
- people who do not respond to treatment.

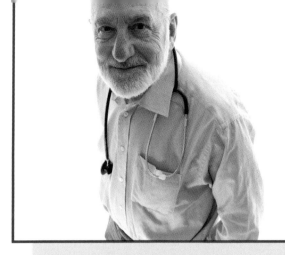

GP

As a GP, I will probably be your first port of call. My role is to recognise and diagnose your bowel complaint and to start the management process. This can mean offering advice and reassurance, recommending lifestyle changes and sometimes prescribing medication, if appropriate. I will ask you about your symptoms and your medical history, and do a physical examination in order to make an accurate diagnosis. If I feel that it is warranted, I can call on specialist opinions from a gastroenterologist or dietitian.

Once your IBS is stabilised, I will work with other members of the healthcare team to ensure that regular reviews and check-ups are arranged for you. These are designed to detect and treat any changes in your IBS, good or bad, and ensure that you get the best possible care. My overall aim is to tailor the management process to suit your individual circumstances. Developing and maintaining long-term relationships with my patients and their families helps me to do this.

MANAGING IBS

Once you have been diagnosed with IBS, your doctor will recommend an appropriate course of treatment. Bear in mind that there is no cure for IBS and that no treatment option is easy. All of them will demand commitment and perseverance on your part. It is also unlikely that the first type of treatment you try will be successful. It will take time and some degree of trial and error to settle on a solution that works best for you.

Your doctor will base any treatment approach on your individual symptoms. Since, as we have seen, one person with IBS is unlikely to complain of exactly the same symptoms as the next, it is easy to see why IBS treatment needs to be individualised. If you suffer from diarrhoea-predominant IBS for example, your doctor will recommend a treatment programme that tackles diarrhoea specifically.

Treatment of IBS can take various forms. It may involve:

- changing your lifestyle
- taking medication
- trying a complementary or alternative therapy
- a mixture of any of the above.

Someone to listen to you

For many people, the relief of learning what's wrong and the reassurance that it's not life-threatening is all the treatment that's needed. If symptoms are mild and don't bother you too much, you may be more inclined to put up with them once you have been given appropriate reassurance.

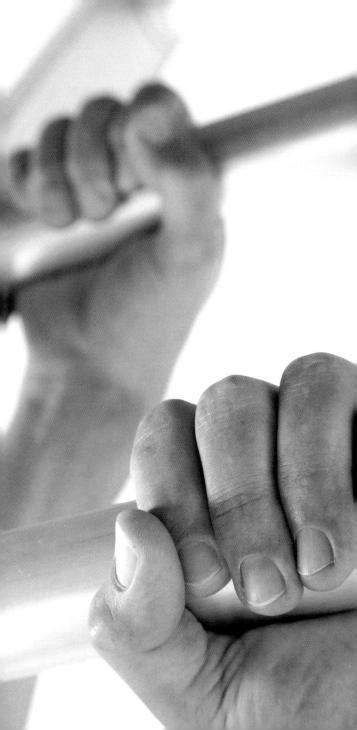

Lifestyle changes

More often than not, your doctor will recommend that you change aspects of your lifestyle in order to improve your IBS symptoms. This usually involves eating a healthy balanced diet. Changing your eating patterns and sometimes cutting out foods that aggravate your symptoms (e.g. dairy products, wheat, potatoes and spicy foods) may minimise the impact IBS has on your life.

Other lifestyle measures, like giving up smoking, cutting down on the amount of alcohol you drink and getting enough sleep can all help. One of the most helpful things you can do is to reduce your stress levels. Your doctor will be able to advise you how best to do this.

THE DIFFERENT DRUGS USED TO TREAT IBS

	Drug class
Drugs used to relieve abdominal pain	Antimuscarinics
	Direct muscle relaxants
	Antidepressants*
Drugs used to treat diarrhoea	Antimotility drugs
Drugs used to treat constipation	Bulk-forming laxatives

* If your doctor prescribes you an antidepressant, it does not mean that he thinks your IBS symptoms are 'all in your head'. At low doses, drugs like amitriptyline act as painkillers rather than antidepressants.

Drug treatment of IBS

Medication may not always be the best option for managing IBS. People with mild symptoms often get more benefit from simply adjusting their lifestyle and trying to de-stress. However, for people with severe symptoms which incapacitate them on a regular basis, drug treatment may help.

Different types of drug treat different elements of IBS, and can be broadly classed as:

■ those that relieve abdominal pain

■ those used to treat diarrhoea

■ those used to treat constipation.

Generic name	Brand name(s)
Hyoscine	Buscopan®
Dicycloverine	Merbentyl®
Alverine	Spasmonal®
Mebeverine	Colofac®, Colofac® MR
Peppermint oil	Colpermin®, Mintec®
Imipramine	Tofranil®
Trimipramine	Surmontil®
Amitriptyline	
Loperamide	Imodium®, Diareze®, Diacalm®
Co-phenotrope	Lomotil®
Codeine	Kaodene®
Ispaghula husk	Fibrelief®, Fybogel®, Isogel®, Ispagel Orange®, Regulan®
Methylcellulose	Celevac®
Sterculia	Normacol®, Normacol Plus®

Complementary and alternative therapies

Many people with IBS also show improvement after:

- hypnotherapy
- relaxation therapy
- biofeedback
- acupuncture
- colonic irrigation.

These techniques are described in more detail later on (see *Managing irritable bowel syndrome* page 106).

Coping with IBS

The best way to manage IBS is to understand it properly. Learning about your body – how it works and what happens when it goes wrong – can help you to get a grip on your symptoms. Of course, reading this book is a great start! Remember, YOU know your body better than anyone else. If you have IBS:

- try not to be embarrassed
- find other sufferers and share your experiences
- don't give up!

If, in partnership with your doctor, you manage your IBS effectively then there is no reason why you can't:

- enjoy going out with friends
- enjoy and perform well at work or school.

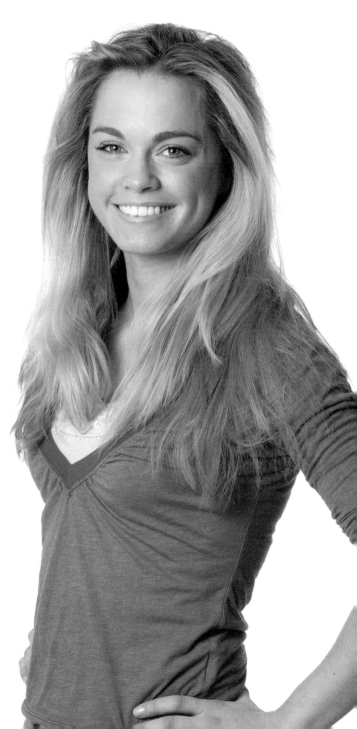

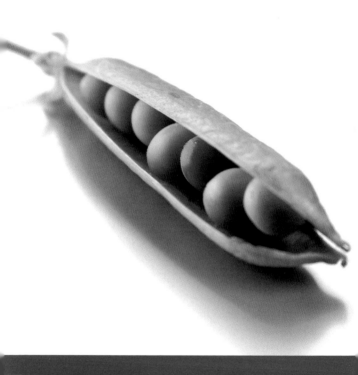

Why me?

WHY ME?

Around 12 million people in the UK have occasional symptoms of IBS, yet over half choose not to report them to their GP. Although it is not life-threatening, IBS is a real medical condition and should be regarded as such, by patients and doctors alike.

HOW COMMON IS IBS?

IBS is the most common disorder of the digestive system with conservative estimates suggesting that it affects between 15 and 20% of the UK population. So, if up to 12 million people in the UK have IBS – why are we not more aware of it?

The answer is simple. The majority of people with IBS have relatively mild symptoms that will come and go, and in all probability will not bother them enough to the extent that they seek out medical advice. Many people don't recognise the symptoms of IBS for what they are and put them down to a bout of food poisoning or simply an 'off' day or two. The embarrassing nature of the symptoms also means that people are reluctant to talk openly about them, to their doctor or anyone else.

Yet despite the fact that most people with IBS never seek medical attention, it is still the most common gastrointestinal problem seen by GPs in the UK. This speaks volumes about the real incidence of IBS and suggests that the actual number of people who are affected is likely to have been grossly underestimated.

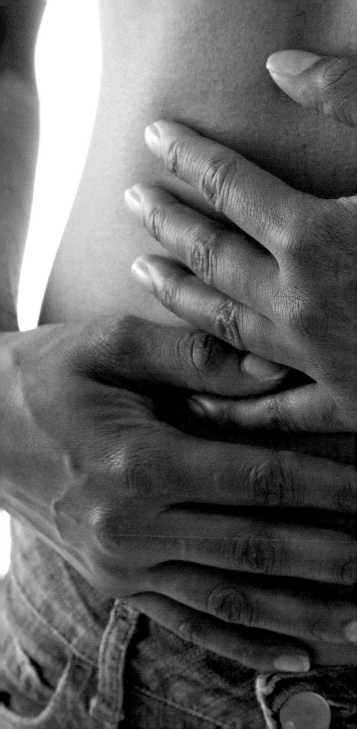

WHO GETS IBS?

The secrecy that surrounds IBS can make it difficult to tell exactly who is affected. Some surveys have reported that up to twice as many women as men have IBS, yet others would dispute that the difference was this large. This disparity probably arises because women are more likely, in general, to seek medical attention for their symptoms than men.

There is generally no difference between men and women in terms of how severe symptoms get, but the nature of symptoms may differ slightly. For example, women are more likely to suffer from bloating and incomplete emptying of the bowels than men. Many women notice that their symptoms become worse around the time when they are having their period.

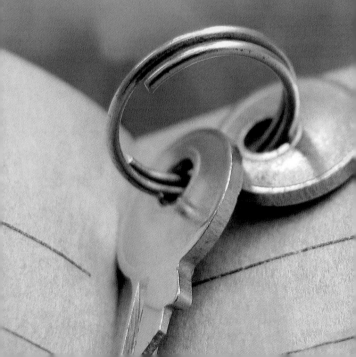

People with IBS generally tend to first notice their symptoms at a relatively young age, with most people who are newly diagnosed with IBS going to see their doctor before they reach 45. That is not to say that older people don't get IBS, but the incidence in this age group is comparatively low. For many people, the symptoms of IBS will resolve, or at least improve, given time.

- Around half of people with IBS first develop symptoms before the age of 35.

- Forty per cent of people with IBS are aged between 35 and 50.

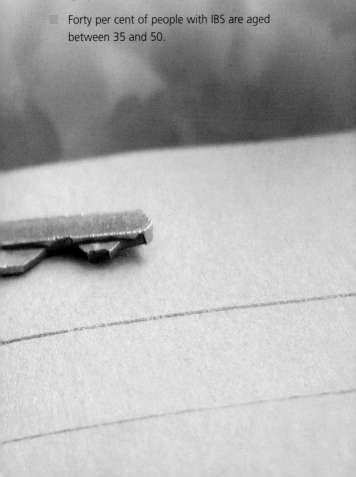

IBS AND QUALITY OF LIFE

Quality of life can be a difficult thing to put a value on. Scientists often use specially designed questionnaires to rate how badly a disease or condition affects a person's ability to get on with their day-to-day life. Whilst these assessments can prove useful, it is often difficult to sum up the impact that IBS has on your life by simply ticking a few boxes.

Still, there is no doubt that IBS can have a significant effect on your day-to-day life. IBS is by nature an unpredictable and personal condition but no-one knows better than you how much of a burden the symptoms of IBS can be. Depending on how severe your symptoms are at any one point in time, IBS can mean that you:

- take a lot of time off work

- miss a lot of school or university

- have to allow extra time to commute to work or school

- avoid making long journeys

- plan your day around the bathroom

- make excuses to avoid social occasions

- constantly have to watch what you eat

- have an erratic and often compromised sex life.

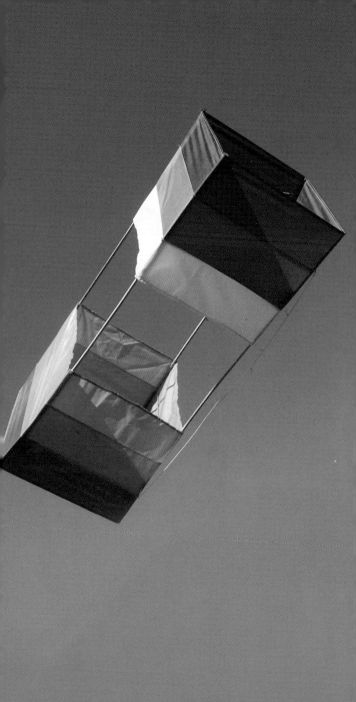

IBS and the workplace

IBS is one of the front runners when it comes to workplace absenteeism, and is only beaten by complaints like the common cold. IBS symptoms often mean people take more time off work or arrive late on a daily basis. Indeed, for many, the working day begins extraordinarily early so that they allow themselves extra time to get to work if their symptoms should worsen suddenly.

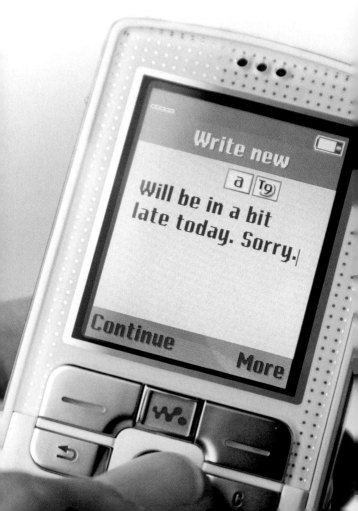

Confiding in your boss can be a daunting prospect, and more often that not, you will not meet with a great deal of sympathy or understanding. For this reason, many people with IBS choose not to tell their boss or other colleagues and are faced with the constant challenge of having to think up excuses for lateness or prolonged absence.

Taking time off work can reduce your chances of a promotion. If your absence is prolonged and seemingly unexplained, it can even place your job at risk. Many people with IBS have admitted to turning down promotion opportunities that would have involved them attending meetings and presentations, and some people have even reported giving up work altogether.

Working in close proximity to other people can amplify the embarrassment factor, so that people with IBS:

■ often aggravate their condition by avoiding using the toilet for as long as possible

■ worry about spending too long in the toilet

■ avoid away days and other social events associated with work

■ often become isolated in the workplace.

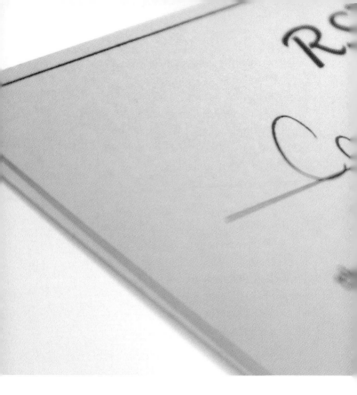

Socialising with IBS

Many people find that they become increasingly isolated from others as a result of their IBS. Constantly having to think up excuses to get out of social occasions can be exhausting and ultimately may end up compromising friendships. Forming new relationships is often made more difficult by IBS. Having to disguise frequent trips to the bathroom, or cancel dates because of abdominal pain, when you are in the early stages of getting to know someone is by no means an easy task.

The best – but certainly not the easiest – approach is to be honest with those around you. Try to educate the people who matter the most to

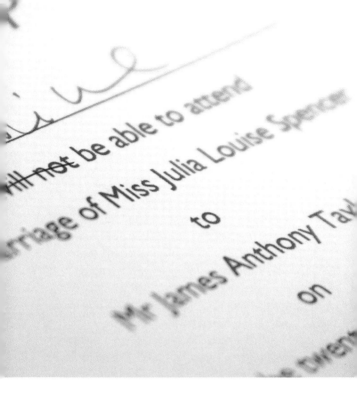

will not be able to attend

...rriage of Miss Julia Louise Spence...

to

Mr James Anthony Tay...

on

...e twen...

you by referring them to books like this one or internet forums. This way they will learn to take your IBS seriously and realise that it is no laughing matter.

Speaking to someone who knows exactly what you're going through can make life much easier. This doesn't just mean your doctor, who is often pushed for time. Nothing beats talking to someone who has experienced what you're going through. Again internet forums are a good place to get in touch with other people with IBS (see *Simple extras* page 124). Your local doctor's surgery may even run a support group (or should at least be able to put you in touch with one).

HOW DID I END UP WITH IBS?

In many cases the actual cause of IBS is unknown, and it is doubtful that you would have been able to do anything to prevent it. Scientists simply do not know enough about the condition to point the finger at any one particular factor.

Although the causes of IBS vary hugely from one person to the next, the underlying malfunction can usually be traced back to the gastrointestinal tract. In people with IBS, the bowel is more sensitive than usual. This over-sensitivity disturbs the speed at which bowel processes take place, which then sets off the symptoms of IBS. Bowel processes are abnormally slow in those people with constipation-predominant IBS and abnormally rapid in those with diarrhoea-predominant IBS. The source of this different 'pace' may be linked to any of the following factors.

■ IBS may run in your family. Recent evidence has hinted that IBS may, at least in part, be linked to your genetic background. However, scientists believe that although you may be more susceptible to IBS because of your genes, you will not necessarily develop it unless other factors come into play.

■ Some people develop IBS for the first time after a bout of gastroenteritis (known as post-infective IBS).

■ IBS can be brought on by an extremely stressful experience like the death of a relative. This is the point after which many people first notice their symptoms developing. There is also some evidence to suggest that sexual or physical abuse during childhood can make you more likely to develop IBS in later life.

■ Your psychological frame of mind can affect your IBS. People who suffer from anxiety and depression are more likely to report IBS symptoms. Although IBS is not caused by psychological problems, the way that different people respond to their IBS can depend on their frame of mind.

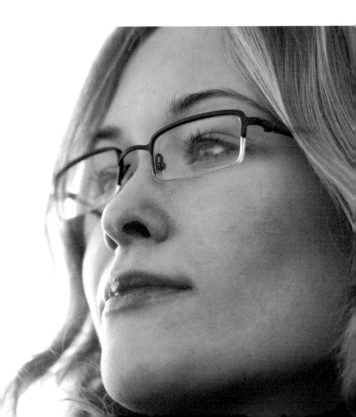

WHAT TRIGGERS IBS?

A trigger is something that worsens or brings on your IBS symptoms, but is not what causes IBS in the first place. It is very difficult to pinpoint a single IBS trigger. Different people attribute their IBS to different things. For example, it may be that a type of food that worsens your symptoms may cause absolutely no ill-effects for another person. Not all people with IBS will relate to the IBS 'triggers' mentioned below, but the chances are that some may strike a chord with you.

■ **Stress**
Stressful situations like trouble at work or marital problems can often trigger an episode of IBS. This may be because stress can cause contractions of the colon in people with IBS.

■ **Certain types of food**
Although actual food allergies are rare in people with IBS, many sufferers see their symptoms worsen after consuming some types of food. This is often referred to as food intolerance. Common culprits are wheat, dairy products, potatoes and onions.

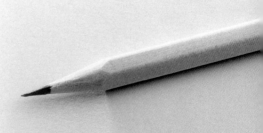

■ **Alcohol**
Certain beers may trigger IBS because a person is sensitive to the levels of yeast contained within them. Cutting down on specific drinks and drinking in moderation can help.

■ **Caffeine**
Tea, coffee and chocolate all contain caffeine, which can open the bowels and cause diarrhoea in people with IBS.

■ **Smoking**
The nicotine in cigarettes acts directly on the muscle of the bowel to make it contract, thereby opening your bowels.

■ **Certain types of medication**
Some types of antibiotics, asthma medications, blood pressure-lowering drugs and painkillers can disrupt digestive processes and may produce IBS symptoms.

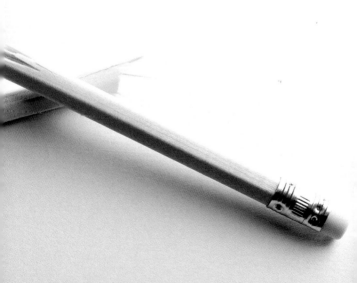

FOOD ALLERGY AND FOOD INTOLERANCE

What's the difference?

Allergy and intolerance are two very different things and should not be confused.

Food allergy is an abnormal response that is triggered by the body's immune system. Eating a food to which you are allergic can cause serious illness and, in some cases, death. In adults, the foods that most often cause allergic reactions include shellfish (such as shrimp, crayfish, lobster and crab), peanuts, tree nuts (such as walnuts), fish and eggs. The symptoms can include rash, itching, swelling, breathing difficulties and even collapse.

Food intolerance is not an allergy because it does not involve the immune system. Although the symptoms can sometimes be similar to those of food allergy (for example, rashes, flushing, abdominal pain, vomiting, diarrhoea and palpitations) they are not usually as severe and food intolerance is rarely life-threatening. Food intolerance is much more common than food allergy. In the UK, most food intolerances involve wheat, dairy products, coffee, potatoes, corn and onions.

People with IBS often notice that eating certain types of food can bring on their symptoms. Remember though, that food intolerance is a result of IBS and not a cause of it.

Types of food intolerance

- Lactose intolerance (inability to digest the sugar found in milk).
- Intolerance to certain preservatives and additives in food (e.g. sulphites, monosodium glutamate (MSG), caffeine and tartrazine; found in canned goods, preserved meats, dairy products and artificially-coloured drinks).
- Food poisoning (e.g. meat contaminated with bacteria).
- Gluten intolerance (inability to digest gluten, the protein found in wheat and some other grains).

Diagnosing food intolerance

Food intolerance is very difficult to diagnose because there are no reliable blood or skin tests that can give a clear 'yes' or 'no' answer. Instead people who suspect they may be unable to tolerate a particular type of food should eliminate it from their diets and see if this makes a difference to their symptoms.

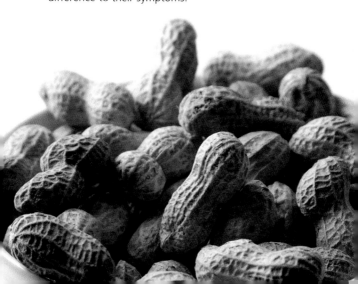

COMMON MISCONCEPTIONS ABOUT IBS

IBS is a disease

FALSE

IBS is not a disease. It is a functional disorder, which means that although the bowel doesn't work as it should, there is no sign of disease when the intestine is examined. Although it can cause considerable pain and discomfort, IBS does not cause lasting damage to the digestive tract, unlike the inflammatory bowel diseases (IBD) Crohn's disease and ulcerative colitis. Crohn's disease and ulcerative colitis are incurable diseases of the gastrointestinal tract. Although they are not usually fatal, they can cause serious problems. Whilst IBD shares many symptoms with IBS (like abdominal pain and diarrhoea), other symptoms (like weight loss, fever, rectal bleeding, loss of appetite) are unique to IBD. No link has been established between IBS and IBD, and having IBS will not make you more likely to develop IBD.

IBS puts you at risk of bowel cancer

FALSE

There is no proven link between IBS and bowel or any other type of cancer. Having IBS will not make you more likely to develop cancer. However, because bowel cancer can sometimes share some symptoms with IBS, your doctor may want to send you for further tests to rule it out. Unlike IBS, cancer rarely causes pain or bloating and its symptoms are not aggravated by eating certain foods.

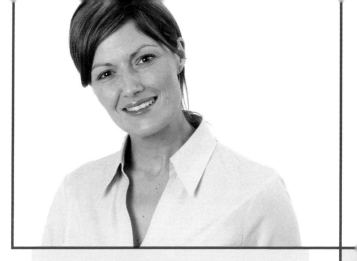

DIETITIAN

As a dietitian I see people referred by their GP or gastroenterologist for dietary advice. Firstly, I will discuss your normal eating habits with you, and work out how your diet ties in with your IBS symptoms. If certain foods (e.g. dairy products, wheat, potatoes and spicy foods) aggravate your IBS, it may be appropriate to exclude these from your diet. These so-called exclusion diets should be closely supervised and this will mean regular follow-up appointments.

There is no hard and fast set of dietary rules that can guarantee success in IBS and for many people it is simply a case of trial and error to work out what is best for them. Keeping a food diary may enable you to identify specific foods that upset you.

I emphasise to all my patients the importance of a healthy balanced diet and the health benefits associated with getting enough fruit and vegetables and eating less saturated fat, salt and sugary foods. Dietary fibre is a contentious issue in IBS and often the best solution is to judge for yourself whether fibre helps or hinders your symptoms and to base any dietary changes on this.

49

IBS is caused by food allergies

FALSE

In fact, as we have seen previously, IBS is rarely linked to food allergy. Although certain types of food can trigger symptoms, this is generally a result of food intolerance rather than true food allergy. Food intolerance is a result and not a cause of IBS.

Less than one bowel movement a day is abnormal

FALSE

Not everyone has a bowel movement every day. It is not abnormal to have as many as three bowel movements a day or as few as three per week.

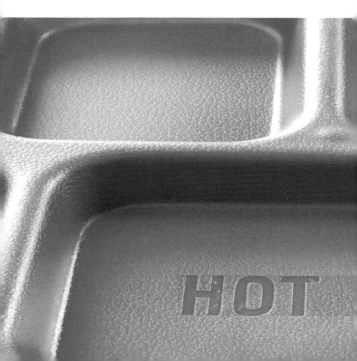

If the pattern of your bowel movements slows down suddenly, it may mean you are getting constipated and if it speeds up then you may experience diarrhoea.

IBS is 'all in the mind'

FALSE

People who have IBS may have a tendency to feel anxious and stressed. But this doesn't mean that IBS is necessarily caused by stress or that the symptoms are all in your mind. IBS is not a psychological or psychiatric disorder but because our gastrointestinal tract is connected to our brain (via the brain–gut axis, see *Simple science* page 56) symptoms can be brought on by stress in some people.

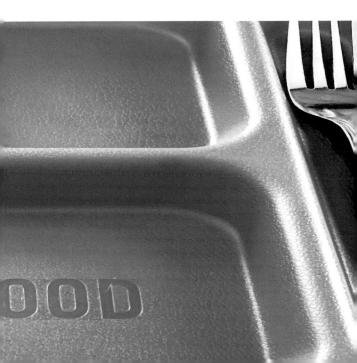

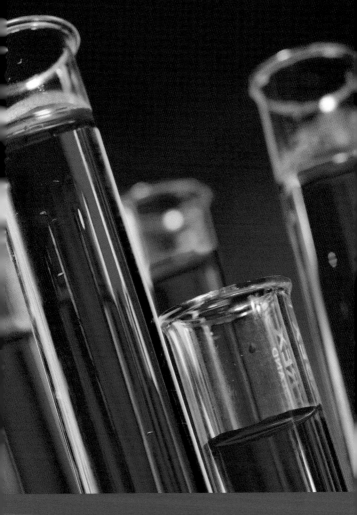

Simple
science

SIMPLE SCIENCE

Learning how your gut should function and what goes wrong when your IBS symptoms flare up can help you to understand your condition and make it easier to live with.

As we have already seen, in people with IBS the function of the gastrointestinal tract changes so that digestion occurs either faster or slower than normal. Although scientists are still trying to pinpoint exactly what happens when you have IBS, they are gradually piecing together the evidence. The three major theories suggest that if you have IBS:

- your gastrointestinal tract is overly sensitive
- the nerves that connect your bowel with your brain function abnormally
- the muscles in the walls of your bowels function abnormally.

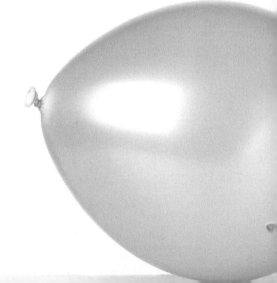

A GUT FEELING

People with IBS may have an oversensitive bowel, which can mean that they react differently to a variety of things, including certain foods and stress. Something that would ordinarily not bother most people (like eating a rich cheese sauce) can prompt a string of symptoms in people with IBS. Pain, discomfort and bloating can be directly linked with having an 'over-reactive' bowel.

This so-called hypersensitivity theory of IBS has been tested in a rather unusual study that involved inserting a balloon-like device into the rectum of 'normal' and 'IBS' volunteers and gradually inflating it. People with IBS became uncomfortable and experienced greater pain at much lower air pressures than those without IBS. People with normally functioning bowels could withstand much greater inflation of the balloon before they noticed any significant pain.

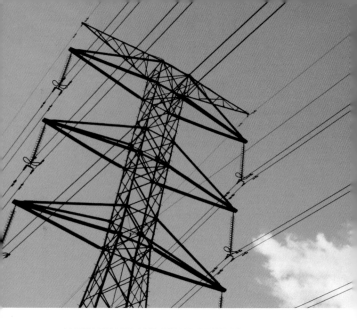

YOUR BRAIN AND YOUR BOWELS

Nerves carry messages between your brain and the muscles in your bowels all the time (a route of communication known as the brain–gut axis). These messages control how fast the bowels work. They also control pain by sending pain signals back to the brain.

It has been suggested that disturbances in the brain–gut axis could account for some of the symptoms of IBS. Indeed, this theory may help to explain why psychological factors like anxiety and stress can trigger the symptoms of IBS.

Nerves that are too active can cause the bowels to expel waste too quickly (diarrhoea). Nerves that aren't active enough can allow waste to stay in the bowels too long (constipation). As we will see later in this section, one of the major substances that helps pass messages between the bowel and brain is called 5-hydroxytryptamine (5-HT, which is also known as serotonin).

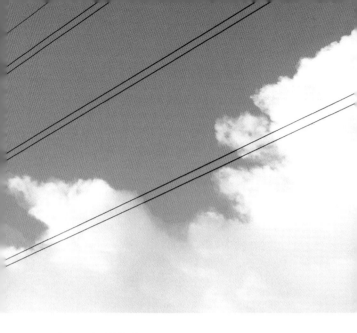

BOWEL MUSCLES

If you have IBS, the muscles controlling your bowels may not work properly. This can affect the motility (muscle movement) of the bowel. If bowel motility is severely affected, the muscles may stop working altogether (albeit temporarily) and constipation can occur.

If bowel motility speeds up (because the bowel muscles are working faster than normal) then this can cause diarrhoea. When bowel muscles go into spasm (sudden, strong muscle contractions that come and go) it can be very unpleasant and this may account for some of the cramping pain associated with IBS.

HOW DO WE TREAT IBS?

Different types of drug treat different aspects of IBS. The treatments that have the greatest impact on the bowel work by either slowing down or speeding up the **transit** of substances through the intestines.

- **Antidiarrhoeals** are medications that slow down intestinal transit. They work by stimulating special receptors (called opiate receptors) in the wall of the bowel and thereby reduce peristalsis (the wave-like process that propels food along the intestine).

- **Laxatives** are medications that speed up intestinal transit. They relieve constipation by forming soft bulky stools and thereby stimulating peristalsis.

A receptor is a docking site on the surface of the wall of the bowel that recognises and attracts a specific chemical messenger, such as a neurotransmitter like serotonin.

Other types of therapy target the brain–gut axis.

■ **Antidepressants** are one such group of drugs. They seem to work by targeting chemicals like serotonin that help pass messages between the bowel and the brain. Chemicals like serotonin are collectively called neurotransmitters. In this way antidepressants may relieve the pain that is associated with IBS (and so are really being used as painkillers rather than antidepressants). They may also increase your sense of well-being (even if you are not depressed in the first place) and help you to cope better with your IBS.

Other drugs help to relieve the pain that is caused by muscle cramping.

■ **Antispasmodics** and **antimuscarinics** help to relax bowel muscle by targeting special receptors located on the bowel muscle itself. These medications can relieve muscle spasm without affecting normal gut motility.

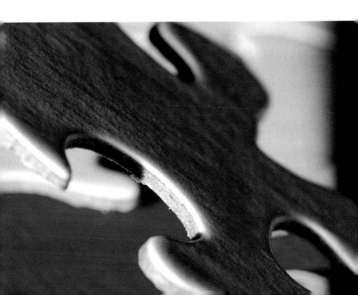

WHAT DOES THE FUTURE HOLD?

Two new types of medication have been developed recently, examples of which are already licensed and being used in the USA. As we went to press they were being reviewed by the licensing authorities for use here in the UK. Both types of medication affect the way that the serotonin neurotransmitter acts on the bowel. Serotonin is thought to be at least partly responsible for a number of important processes in the bowel.

1. Initiating peristalsis.
2. Controlling the secretion of lubricating substances that help with gastrointestinal transit.
3. Controlling the perception of pain.

- **Tegaserod** is a serotonin receptor agonist. This means that it mimics the effects of serotonin in the bowel by targeting the same receptor that serotonin usually targets. In this way, tegaserod enhances peristalsis and stimulates intestinal transit. It can therefore be used to improve symptoms in people with constipation-predominant IBS.

- **Alosetron** and **cilansetron** are serotonin receptor antagonists. This means that they occupy serotonin receptors and stop serotonin from targeting them. In this way they slow down intestinal transit and can therefore be used to improve symptoms in people with diarrhoea-predominant IBS.

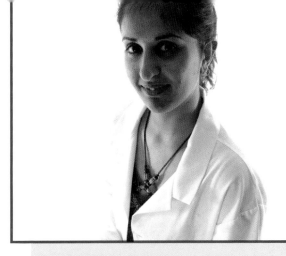

PHARMACIST

As a pharmacist within the Primary Care Trust, I offer people essential services like drug dispensing and self-care support, usually within their local area. I can also provide you with lifestyle advice (such as what to include in a healthy diet).

Pharmacists within the community now play a bigger role than ever before in helping patients to manage their conditions. This may involve keeping track of which medications you are using and how often. A number of new schemes have been laid out in our new pharmacy contract, which reflects the government's health priorities: support for self-care, management of long-term conditions and public health.

By increasing the range of services that we can offer, we can improve the level of care and support that you, as a patient with a long-term condition like IBS, can expect from your health service.

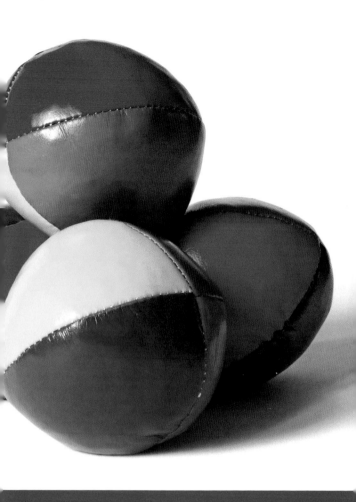

Managing
irritable bowel
syndrome

MANAGING IBS

IBS can be overwhelming and at times it can feel like you will never be able to live a normal life. However, try not to give up hope. It is important to keep looking for possible solutions to the problems your IBS poses.

HOW WILL IBS AFFECT MY LIFE?

The symptoms of IBS are usually unique to each person affected. In reality, it is unlikely that any two people with IBS will suffer from exactly the same range, pattern and intensity of symptoms. This makes it difficult to predict exactly how IBS will affect you. It may be that you experience periods when your IBS disappears and doesn't bother you, but there may also be times when you are bothered by your symptoms more than ever and the outlook seems bleak.

Whatever your particular circumstances, it is a safe bet that IBS has knocked your confidence in some way. The key to managing IBS effectively, lies in your ability to restore your confidence so that you can deal with everything that IBS throws at you.

Always remember, however bad your symptoms get, that IBS is not life-threatening and is not a sign of a more serious underlying condition. Everyone's solution will differ, but with a combination of self-help and possibly medication, it should be possible to prevent IBS from interfering too much with your normal day-to-day life.

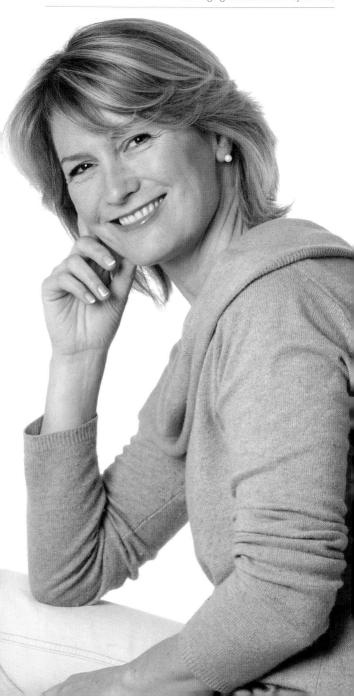

WHEN SHOULD I SEEK MEDICAL HELP?

Although most people find that they are able to manage their IBS without having to visit their GP, if you feel that your symptoms are so severe that they are starting to seriously affect the way you live your life, it is important that you seek medical advice.

Many people with severe IBS choose to continue to suffer in silence and only consult their GP as a last resort. Their reluctance to talk about IBS is understandable. Symptoms can be embarrassing to discuss, and the way in which they come and go can mean that by the time your appointment comes around, you are feeling fine once more. However, since your IBS will most likely rear its head again at some point, it is important to keep your appointment.

Your doctor will be able to:

- help put your mind at rest
- rule out other more serious conditions
- offer you useful advice to help reduce the frequency and severity of your IBS symptoms.

DOS AND DON'TS

- **Don't** leave it until your symptoms become unbearable and your life becomes significantly disrupted before you seek medical help.
- **Don't** assume that your GP will not be able to do anything to help.
- **Do** be prepared to make more than one visit to your GP before you find a solution that works for you.

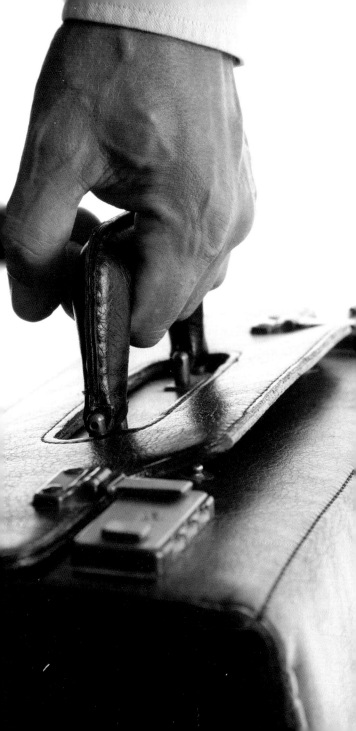

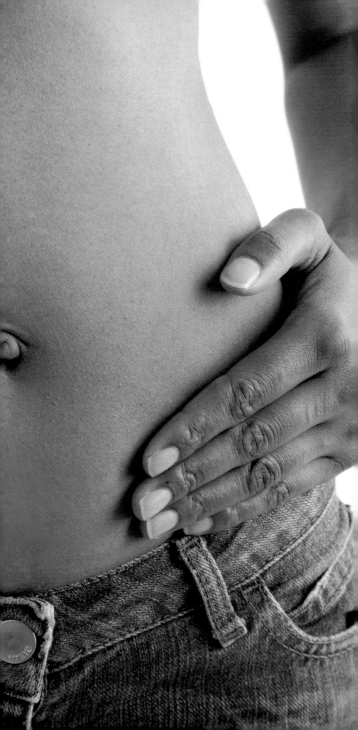

DIAGNOSING IBS

When you first visit your GP, he or she will ask you a number of questions about your symptoms and about your health in general.

- When did you first notice these symptoms?
- Is the pain localised in the same area or does it move around?
- What happens to the pain when you open your bowels?
- How often do you experience bloating?
- How many times do you go to the toilet on a good/bad day?

By taking into account the intensity, timing and location of your pain as you describe it, your doctor will be able to determine whether your symptoms are typical of IBS or whether they may be a sign of another condition.

Your doctor will also consider your age, gender, family medical history and your dietary habits (and how these relate to the onset of your symptoms). Be prepared to answer some personal questions. Your doctor will be trying to establish whether factors like your working environment, relationship difficulties and major life events (like a family bereavement) are contributing to your symptoms.

He or she may also examine your abdomen. This is to make sure there are no swellings or lumps, and no tenderness.

THE ROME II CRITERIA

Doctors sometimes use certain criteria to diagnose IBS. The Rome II criteria specify that people with IBS should have suffered from abdominal pain for 12 consecutive weeks during the past 12 months. The pain should have two of the following three features.

1. It is relieved by having a bowel movement.
2. It is associated with a change in stool frequency.
3. It is associated with a change in the appearance of stools.

Other features can include:

- passing an abnormal number of stools
- passing stools of an abnormal appearance
- passing mucus in the stools
- bloating.

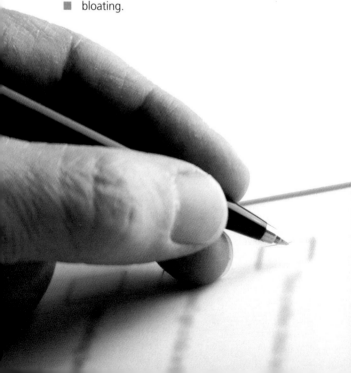

'RED FLAGS'

There are certain symptoms that can alert a doctor to other, potentially more serious, bowel complaints. These so-called 'red flag' symptoms include:

- unexplained weight loss
- a temperature
- passing blood from the back passage
- unexplained masses in the abdomen
- diarrhoea that wakes you from your sleep.

People aged over 45 years who are experiencing symptoms for the first time or people of any age who have a strong history of any type of gastrointestinal cancer in their family, are usually referred to a specialist in order to rule out more serious diseases like colon cancer.

TRUSTING YOUR DOCTOR

Your GP should be able to put aside adequate time for you to discuss your symptoms in some depth. He or she should also listen closely to what you're saying and give you a satisfactory explanation as to why you are experiencing these things and reassure you that your symptoms are not a sign of more serious underlying disease.

What if your doctor has missed something more sinister? A high proportion of people diagnosed with IBS admit that they initially feared that they had colon cancer. It is also fair to say that in many of these people, some element of fear remained even after they had sought a medical opinion. Could your doctor be wrong about your IBS? If they have taken a good history of your symptoms, carried out an appropriate examination and confirmed that any subsequent tests are normal then this is very unlikely.

Although you may not like what your doctor is telling you, trust their experience and judgement. Try to work with them. Having said that, if your doctor is not sympathetic to your concerns, then try another doctor. This is after all your right (see *Simple extras* page 126).

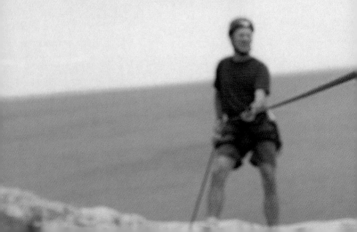

WILL I BE REFERRED?

Most people with IBS can be diagnosed and managed effectively in their family doctor's surgery. However, some people may be referred to a specialist (called a gastroenterologist). Referral may be necessary for:

- people of a certain age (over 45 years)
- people with very severe or constant symptoms
- people with unusual symptoms
- people who do not respond to standard treatments
- people with a history of other more serious gastrointestinal diseases in their family.

Even if your doctor does refer you to a specialist clinic, it doesn't necessarily mean that you have anything more sinister than IBS. In fact, 20–50% of people referred to gastroenterology clinics are diagnosed with IBS in the end.

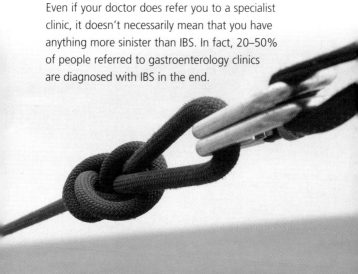

LOOKS LIKE IBS BUT COULD IT BE SOMETHING ELSE?

Other diseases and disorders share some symptoms with IBS and include:

- inflammatory bowel disease or IBD (e.g. Crohn's disease, ulcerative colitis)
- malabsorption diseases (e.g. coeliac disease)
- gastrointestinal infection
- gynaecological disorders (e.g. premenstrual syndrome, endometriosis)
- bowel (or colon) cancer
- hormonal disorders (e.g. thyroid disorders).

When you first report your symptoms to your doctor, they will try to exclude other diseases by asking you a number of questions and will sometimes recommend that you undergo further tests.

TESTING FOR IBS

Although there is no specific test that can be used to diagnose IBS, your GP or specialist may recommend that certain tests are performed. This is simply a precautionary measure that is used to rule out other diseases.

- **Blood tests**

  These can show whether you have an infection in your bowels or if you have anaemia (reduced levels of iron in your blood). Blood tests can also help to rule out other types of bowel disease, like Crohn's disease and coeliac disease. The levels of certain hormones in your bloodstream may also indicate a thyroid disorder, which can share some symptoms with IBS.

■ Analysis of a stool sample

Like blood tests, laboratory tests on stool samples can also be used to confirm infections and to check for small quantities of blood.

■ Food intolerance tests

Rarely, IBS can be related to intolerance of certain types of foods. A simple breath test can reveal whether you are intolerant to lactose (the sugar found in milk and other dairy products).

■ Sigmoidoscopy

An instrument called a sigmoidoscope (a camera attached to a flexible tube) is inserted into the rectum to closely examine the lining of the bowel to identify any abnormalities.

■ Colonoscopy

A similar procedure to sigmoidoscopy that examines the whole of the bowel and is usually performed under sedation.

■ Barium enema

Barium, a chalky substance, is used to partially fill and open up the colon. This allows an X-ray of the colon to be taken, and can be used to exclude cancer and other serious diseases.

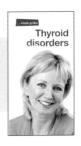

For more information see
Thyroid disorders

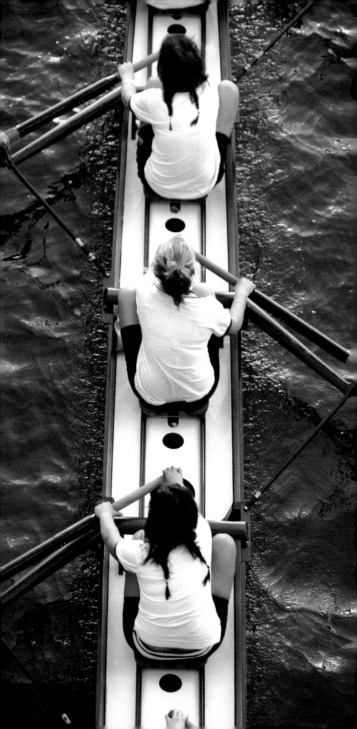

TAKING CONTROL OF YOUR IBS

Controlling your IBS is all about identifying a personal management strategy. This may mean:

- modifying your lifestyle
- changing your diet
- controlling your stress
- taking medications
- trying complementary or alternative therapies.

Be prepared to try each management strategy in turn, as well as a combination of all of them. It will take time to recognise which strategy is most effective. Always remember that the best placed person to judge what works best for you is YOU.

- Remember that you know your body better than anyone else.
- The more you learn about IBS, the easier it will be to manage it. Gather and read as much information about IBS as you can. Of course, reading this book is a great start!
- Consult your GP about your symptoms – it's what they are there for!
- Take an active role in the management programme your doctor devises for you and ask lots of questions during your consultations – this is YOUR time.
- Use patient forums on the internet to exchange information about IBS.
- Communicate with other IBS sufferers and share your experiences with them. Being aware that you're not the only one with a problem can be immensely reassuring and encouraging.
- Try not to be embarrassed about your IBS. Don't give up hope.

LIFESTYLE CHANGES

If you have been diagnosed with IBS, one of the first things that your doctor will ask you to do is to change certain aspects of lifestyle. You will probably need to experiment with the various lifestyle changes mentioned below before you experience any kind of relief. Lifestyle changes may include:

- changing certain aspects of your diet

- cutting out caffeine

- giving up smoking

- de-stressing your life

- exercising regularly

- allowing adequate time for regular defecation

- changing your outlook on life.

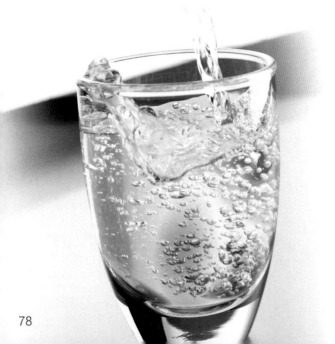

IBS and diet

With IBS, changing your eating habits can be a very hit and miss business. What works well for one person may do nothing for another, and in some instances may even aggravate symptoms. There is no hard and fast set of dietary rules that can guarantee success in IBS and for many people it is simply a case of trial and error to work out what is best for them. Keeping a food diary may enable you to identify specific foods that upset you. The importance of eating a healthy, balanced diet cannot be overstated.

Controlling IBS is not just about the types of food you eat but also how you eat them. Making some of the following changes to your eating habits may help to improve your IBS symptoms:

- eat slowly in a relaxed environment

- allow yourself enough time to eat (at least 20 minutes per meal)

- chew food well and relax before and after eating in an upright position

- eat regularly (at least three times a day) and space meals at regular intervals

- eat smaller portions (but more frequently)

- do not over eat, especially just before you go to bed

- drink plenty of fluids (preferably water).

Dietary fibre

Fibre (or roughage) is a contentious issue in IBS. Many experts have conflicting opinions and as yet have failed to come up with a definitive answer on the fibre question. So what is dietary fibre and how does it affect digestion?

Fibre is the framework of a plant, the part that holds it together and keeps it structurally sound. As a food substance, it is therefore extremely difficult to digest. It can withstand chewing and the highly acidic and hostile conditions of the stomach to emerge from our bodies virtually unchanged. Although it is difficult to break down and use as a source of energy, fibre is nonetheless essential for maintaining bowel health, largely because it:

- increases the weight of faeces
- speeds up bowel processes
- increases the number of bowel movements.

There are two types of fibre, soluble and insoluble. Soluble fibre (found in fruits, vegetables, pulses, oats and barley) dissolves in water and forms gels that help to stabilise blood sugar levels and reduce the amount of cholesterol absorbed from the intestine (thereby helping to protect us against things like heart disease). Insoluble fibre (found in fruits and vegetables with skins and pips, wheat, rye, rice and nuts) does not dissolve and instead holds on to water. This adds weight and bulk to the faeces and helps waste pass through the bowel more easily. It also helps to protect the bowel against disease.

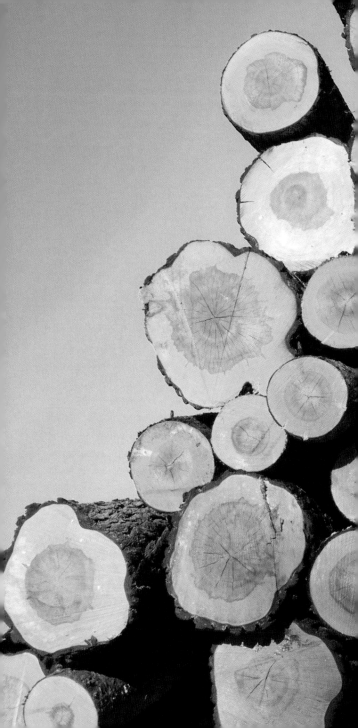

There are three main ways you can increase your intake of fibre.

1. Follow a healthy natural high-fibre diet (i.e. one which is rich in fruits and vegetables).

2. Eat fibre-rich foods (whole-wheat cereals, wholemeal bread and brown rice).

3. Take fibre supplements in the form of bran and bulk-forming laxatives.

It is easy to understand why fibre may have a key role to play in IBS. Whether or not increasing the amount of fibre that you eat actually helps to reduce your symptoms, is largely dependent on the type of IBS that you suffer from. The people who gain the most benefit from increasing their fibre intake are generally those who suffer from constipation-predominant and mixed type IBS. Because fibre accelerates the transit of food substances through the bowel, it can help to speed up this process and relieve the painful constipation that afflicts these people. Conversely, rapid transit through the bowel is one of the major problems underlying diarrhoea-predominant IBS and so further accelerating the process will only aggravate symptoms and make the situation worse.

The best solution is to judge for yourself whether fibre helps or hinders your IBS symptoms and to base any dietary changes on this.

Exclusion diets

If you have IBS you will be well aware that if you eat certain foods you will usually end up regretting it. This may be linked to food intolerance (see *Why me?* page 46). Like most things linked to IBS, food triggers are varied and are often unique to each individual person.

Because certain symptoms of IBS can be strongly aggravated by specific foods, it may actually make sense to rule them out of your diet completely. However, these so-called exclusion or elimination diets may not always be the best thing for you. Be careful that you don't end up ruling out too many different foods to the extent that your diet is drastically compromised. Eliminating key food types can mean that you lose out on essential nutrients. Strict exclusion diets have very low success rates in IBS and can sometimes do more harm than good.

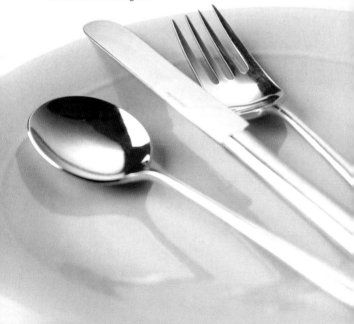

Probiotics

These days, supermarket shelves are crammed with probiotic supplements like Yakult®, Actimel®, Danone® and Proviva®. Although clinical studies of probiotics have so far only involved relatively small groups of people, emerging evidence suggests that they may help to improve the symptoms of IBS.

We all have bacteria living in our gastrointestinal tracts. These 'gut microflora' produce essential nutrients, help to manufacture vitamins and protect us against potentially harmful bacteria. Using these friendly gut microflora (or 'probiotics') as food supplements is based on the assumption that introducing extra 'healthy' bacteria into our bodies will improve our digestive health by re-balancing the levels of bacteria within our intestines. This is not a new idea. The health benefits associated with introducing strains of live bacteria into foods was recognised as long ago as 1905, by a Russian scientist called Élie Metchnikoff.

The next few years will probably yield significant findings in the area of probiotics. It is possible that in the future, more powerful probiotics will be available from your doctor on a prescription-only basis. The concentration of active ingredients will be much higher than that found in the commercial products currently available in supermarkets.

Prebiotics

Snapping at the heels of the probiotics are the prebiotics. Rather than introducing additional bacteria into the body like the probiotics, the prebiotics work by feeding up the good bacteria that already exist in the digestive tract and helping them to function more effectively. It is likely that we'll be hearing a lot more about prebiotics in the near future.

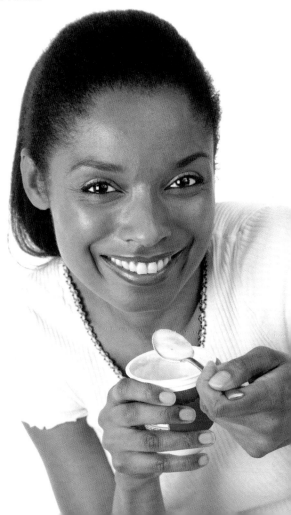

IBS AND THE FOOD YOU EAT

- Be prepared to make 'food mistakes' and make sure you learn from them.

- Always try to eat a healthy balanced diet.

- Experiment with the amount of fibre you eat. See what works best for you.

- Probiotics can help to restore the balance of bacteria in your digestive system and may improve your symptoms – give them a try.

- Exclude with caution. Cutting an essential food type out of your diet can sometimes do more harm than good. Make sure you seek advice from your doctor before trying this.

- Do everything gradually to give you body time to adjust. Don't expect quick fixes.

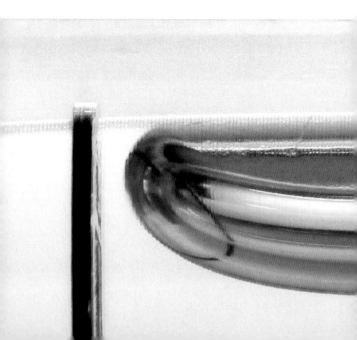

If you do make changes to your diet make sure that you do it gradually so that your body has time to adjust. Also make sure that you seek professional advice from your GP before embarking on anything too drastic.

Try keeping a food diary of exactly what you eat and how it ties in with your IBS to try to identify exactly which foods are triggering your symptoms. You may find that cutting down on some of the following foods helps:

- dairy products
- spicy foods
- cereals
- foods that contain high quantities of sorbitol (a sugar found naturally in apricots, cherries and apples)
- caffeine.

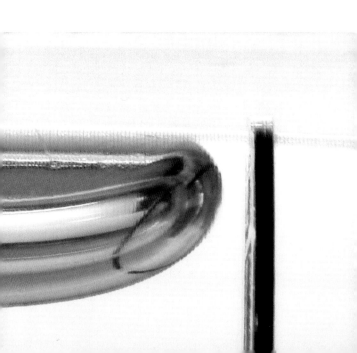

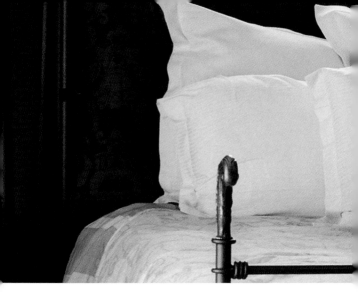

STRESS

Recognising that stress can trigger your IBS is only half the battle. De-stressing is the other half. Constantly worrying about work, family or relationship problems, exams and financial difficulties will take its toll on your digestive tract, especially if you are susceptible to IBS in the first place. The worry that IBS itself brings with it, only helps to fuel this self-perpetuating circle of stress. Your GP may be able to suggest ways in which you can deal with stress effectively, without having to resort to drug treatment. Learning relaxation techniques (see page 109) and speaking to a stress counsellor may help you to control your symptoms.

Whilst smoking may be something that you resort to in times of stress, its important to try to give up. Aside from the detrimental effects smoking has on your general health, the nicotine

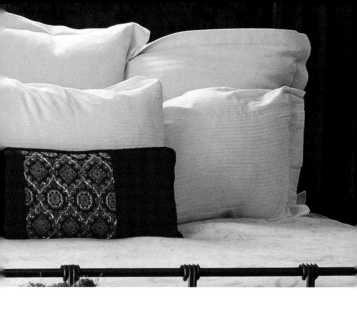

in cigarettes acts directly on intestinal muscle and makes it contract, thereby opening your bowels. This can sometimes be the last thing you want if you have IBS.

The power of getting a good night's sleep should also not be underestimated. Many people with IBS notice that their symptoms worsen considerably the morning after a night of interrupted sleep. Improve your sleep pattern by:

- cutting down on caffeine, nicotine or alcohol close to bedtime
- avoiding heavy meals close to bedtime
- taking a warm bath
- exercising regularly
- making your bedroom a nice place to be
- trying relaxation and deep breathing techniques.

EXERCISE

On bad days, exercise may well be the last thing that you feel like doing. Yet it may be worth forcing yourself. Many people with IBS experience some form of relief from their symptoms by taking regular exercise.

- Exercising is a good way of taking your mind off your IBS.

- Exercise is a fantastic 'de-stressor'.

- The endorphins (natural pain-killers) you produce when you exercise can make you feel better.

- Exercise helps you to stay in shape, and staying in shape increases your confidence and self-esteem, something that IBS may have dented.

- Exercise can improve the quality of your sleep.

- Exercising can reduce muscle tension (this goes for all muscles, including the ones in your digestive system).

- Moderate exercise boosts your immune system and can make you less susceptible to illness.

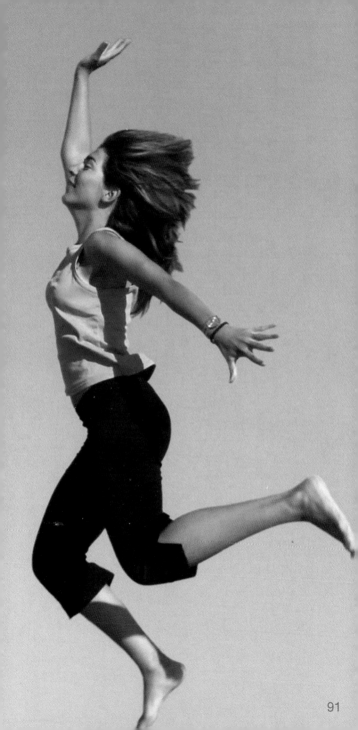

CHANGING YOUR OUTLOOK

Last but not least, changing the way that you view your IBS can improve your symptoms quite dramatically. Do not let IBS rule your life. Think positive. Try to slow down and make the time to look after yourself properly. Simple things, like allowing enough time to go to the toilet without having to rush, can be surprisingly effective.

Bear in mind that you are unlikely to hit upon a perfect solution straight away. Discovering what works best for you can be hit and miss and some degree of perseverance is required. Do your own research; ask other people with IBS what they find works for them. Don't be afraid to keep going back to see your GP, especially if your symptoms worsen or change suddenly, this after all is what they're there for.

How to ensure your toilet is a nice place to be

- Keep it clean

- Keep it warm

- Keep it fragrant

- Keep it relaxed – music can help to create a relaxing atmosphere

- Keep it well stocked – toilet paper should be in abundance

- Keep it private – make sure the lock works!

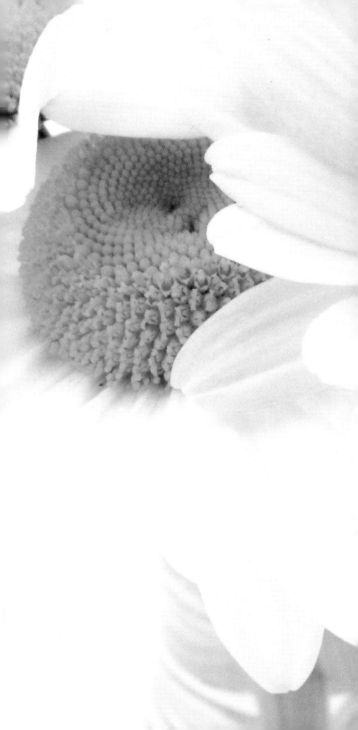

CONTROLLING IBS WITH DRUG TREATMENT

When you are first diagnosed with IBS, your doctor may not prescribe you a course of drug treatment straight away. This is because often, people with IBS respond well to simple lifestyle changes (like those mentioned earlier in this section) and there is no need for them to take medication, except perhaps on an occasional basis.

Your doctor will usually only prescribe you drug treatment if changing your lifestyle has failed to improve your symptoms as well as they would have hoped, or if your symptoms are particularly severe.

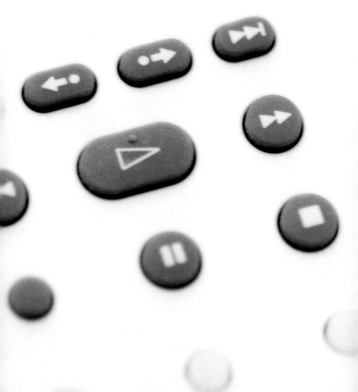

If you are prescribed medication, it is important to remember that you may not notice a drastic improvement in your IBS symptoms straight away. As with the lifestyle changes discussed previously, there is a certain amount of trial and error when it comes to selecting the best drug treatment for your individual circumstances. Drug treatment for IBS:

■ may not work for everyone, some people may respond well but others may not notice any difference in their symptoms

■ is sometimes associated with unpleasant side-effects (see page 102)

■ may treat one type of symptom but make no impression on others

■ may not be as successful as some lifestyle or dietary changes.

Drugs are usually reserved for those people with 'moderate or severe' IBS. People with mild symptoms do not usually need medication to manage their IBS effectively.

WHICH DRUGS WILL I BE PRESCRIBED?

If you do qualify for drug treatment, your doctor will base your treatment around your predominant IBS symptom, be it constipation, diarrhoea, or a mixture of the two. This is because the different types of drugs used to treat IBS have different targets within the body. Each drug treats an individual symptom of IBS. It would make no sense to give a person with constipation-predominant IBS an anti-diarrhoeal, for example. Bear in mind that many of the drugs listed below are generally reserved for people with more severe IBS that has not responded to alternative, non-drug treatment approaches.

In order to help them tailor your drug treatment to your personal set of symptoms, doctors use specially constructed guidelines to decide on a treatment approach. In the UK, these guidelines are published by the Primary Care Society for Gastroenterology (*www.pcsg.org.uk*).

Tegaserod, alosetron and cilansetron are new drugs that may soon be available in the UK for the treatment of IBS (see *Simple science* page 60).

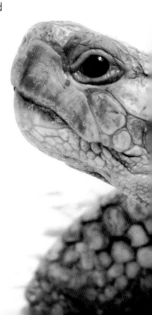

The drugs and medications referred to in this Simple Guide are believed to be currently in widespread use in the UK. Medical science can evolve rapidly, but to the best of our knowledge, this is a reasonable reflection of clinical practice at the time of going to press.

Source: British National Formulary.

DRUGS USED TO TREAT DIARRHOEA

Medications that are used to treat diarrhoea generally work by reducing the number of bowel movements you have. They are also known as antimotility drugs. Such drugs include:

- loperamide (Imodium®, Diareze®, Diacalm®)

- co-phenotrope (Lomotil®)

- codeine (Kaodene®).

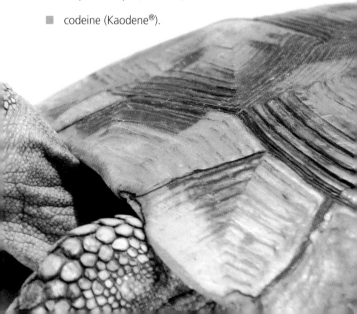

DRUGS USED TO TREAT CONSTIPATION

In contrast to antidiarrhoeals, drugs that are used to relieve the constipation that is associated with IBS (often called laxatives) increase the number of bowel movements you have. Usually, eating a balanced diet that includes adequate fibre and drinking plenty of liquids is enough to prevent constipation. You can also boost your intake of dietary fibre by taking bran supplements. Your doctor will only recommend a laxative if your bowel movements are very infrequent and vary significantly from your normal routine. Taking laxatives unnecessarily can do more harm than good and they are open to abuse by people with eating disorders or those hoping to lose weight rapidly. Laxatives are not generally used in children, other than in exceptional circumstances.

Bulk-forming laxatives like ispaghula husk (Fibrelief®, Fybogel®, Isogel®, Ispagel Orange® and Regulan®), methylcellulose (Celevac®) and sterculia (Normacol® and Normacol Plus®) can be used to treat the constipation that is sometimes associated with IBS.

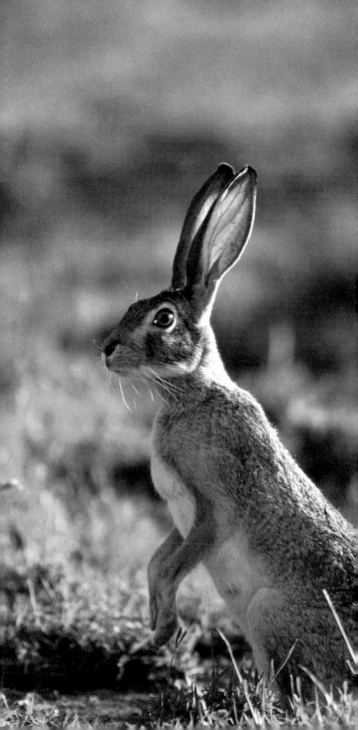

DRUGS USED TO TREAT ABDOMINAL PAIN

As we have mentioned previously, pain is often the most unpleasant symptom of IBS and the symptom that most often drives people to seek medical help. There are a number of different medications that can be used to relieve the pain associated with IBS.

Since most IBS pain is caused by the gastrointestinal muscle going into spasm, drugs which help to relax the muscle can offer pain relief. These include:

- antimuscarinics (e.g. hyoscine [Buscopan®], dicycloverine [Merbentyl®])
- direct muscle relaxants (e.g. alverine [Spasmonal®], mebeverine [Colofac®] and peppermint oil [Colpermin®, Mintec®]).

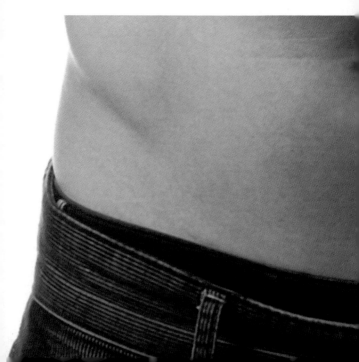

Other drugs that can relieve the pain and muscle spasm associated with IBS include:

- antidepressants (e.g. amitriptyline, imipramine [Tofranil®], trimipramine [Surmontil®]).

It may seem strange to treat IBS with the same drugs that are used to treat depression, especially if you are not depressed in the first place. If your doctor prescribes you an antidepressant, it does not mean that he thinks your IBS symptoms are 'all in your head'. No-one knows exactly why antidepressants offer benefit against IBS, but the fact remains that they CAN work. The doses of these drugs prescribed for IBS are much lower than those used to treat depression. At low doses, drugs like amitriptyline act as painkillers rather than antidepressants.

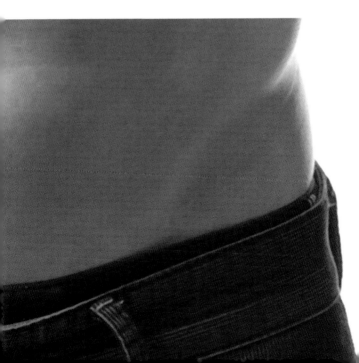

THE SIDE-EFFECTS MOST OFTEN ASSOCIATED WITH IBS MEDICATIONS

Drug type	Possible side-effects
Antimuscarinics	Constipation, palpitations, urinary urgency and retention, blurred vision, dry mouth, flushing and dryness of the skin.
Direct muscle relaxants	Nausea, headache, rash and dizziness. Heartburn has also been linked with peppermint oil.
Antidepressants	Drowsiness, dry mouth, blurred vision, constipation, urinary retention and heart arrhythmias.
Antimotility drugs	Nausea, vomiting, constipation, dizziness and drowsiness. Larger doses can affect breathing and cause low blood pressure, produce respiratory depression and hypotension (low blood pressure).
Laxatives	Flatulence, bloating and swelling of the abdomen.

No drug treatment is without side-effects, and different people may respond in slightly different ways to the same medicine. If you experience symptoms which you think may be due to the medication you are taking, you should talk to your doctor, pharmacist or nurse. If the side-effect is unusual or severe, your GP may decide to report it to the Medicines and Healthcare products Regulatory Agency (MHRA). The MHRA operates a 'Yellow Card Scheme' which is designed to flag up potentially dangerous drug effects and thereby protect your safety. The procedure has changed recently to allow patients to report adverse drug reactions themselves. Visit *www.yellowcard.gov.uk* for more information. You should always ask your doctor if you are concerned about any aspect of your IBS management plan.

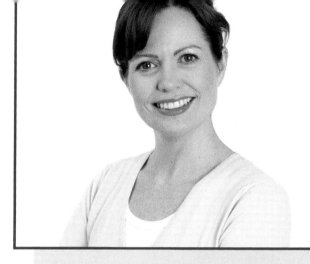

THERAPIST

There are many types of complementary and alternative medicine that can benefit people with IBS. Hypnotherapy, relaxation therapy, cognitive behavioural therapy, biofeedback and psychotherapy have all proved successful in certain people.

These techniques use a variety of approaches, from visualising a healthy digestive system to understanding how your body should be working and recognising when things start to go wrong. Most of these therapies help you to reduce your stress levels and release tension in your body. Cognitive behavioural therapy can help to improve your IBS symptoms by breaking them down into manageable parts, working out how they are connected and seeing how they ultimately affect you.

As a therapist, I will have specialised in a particular area. I usually work in collaboration with the primary care team, and am sometimes based at the GP surgery itself. Although most of these techniques are widely available, in some instances it may be difficult to locate a specialist in your local area. Your GP will usually be able to advise you.

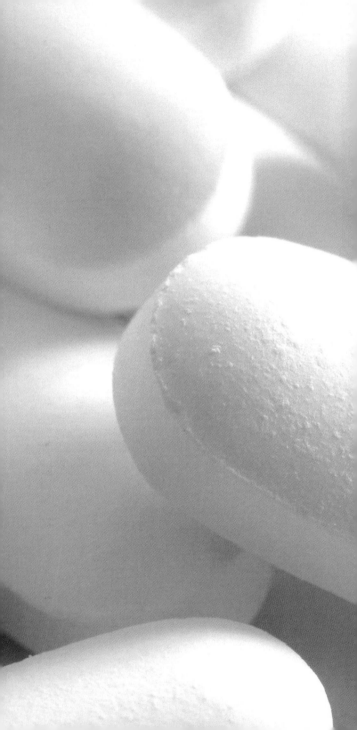

IBS AND THE PLACEBO EFFECT

A placebo is something that looks like a drug (in terms of its size, colour and shape) but has no actual medicinal value. Placebos are used in clinical trials to determine whether any drug or treatment will be effective. If those trial participants who are taking the placebo respond in the same way as those taking the active drug, then the active drug is not particularly effective!

Sometimes, people respond very well to treatment with a placebo, even though it contains no active ingredient. This is called a 'placebo effect' and is linked to the way in which our minds respond to the physical act of taking a 'drug'. If a person (or indeed their doctor) has high hopes and believes in a treatment, the chances are they will gain some kind of benefit from it, even though it may not be due to anything a drug is doing. Put simply, the patient wants the drug to work so they perceive that it does.

In IBS, the placebo effect can be very strong (although this does not mean that IBS is all 'in the mind'). Between 40 and 70% of people receiving treatment for IBS will improve with placebo alone. The placebo effect usually wears off after a few weeks and so it is not a long-term solution.

COMPLEMENTARY AND ALTERNATIVE THERAPIES

Hypnotherapy

Although some people may be sceptical, hypnotherapy is actually a well-established treatment for IBS and can work very well for some people. Having said that, hypnotherapy is a very expensive treatment and is often time-consuming – requiring up to 12 half-hourly sessions before any improvement is observed. If you are considering a course of hypnotherapy, it is vital that you use a reputable hypnotherapist. The UK Hypnotherapy Society (*www.hypnotherapysociety.com*) should be able to put you in touch with someone in your local area.

So how does hypnotherapy work? Relatively little is known about exactly what makes hypnosis so effective for IBS. Many experts believe it is the state of relaxation that hypnosis induces that is responsible. A relaxed mind is open to suggestions and new ideas. After inducing hypnosis, the hypnotherapist may ask you to visualise a healthy digestive system or other bowel-directed positive imagery. This forms the basis for the whole technique. Patients are often given a short audiotape of home exercises to supplement their course of treatment.

The benefits of a course of hypnosis can last for as long as 2 years after treatment has finished. All major IBS symptoms (including pain, diarrhoea, constipation and bloating) can show improvement after this kind of treatment.

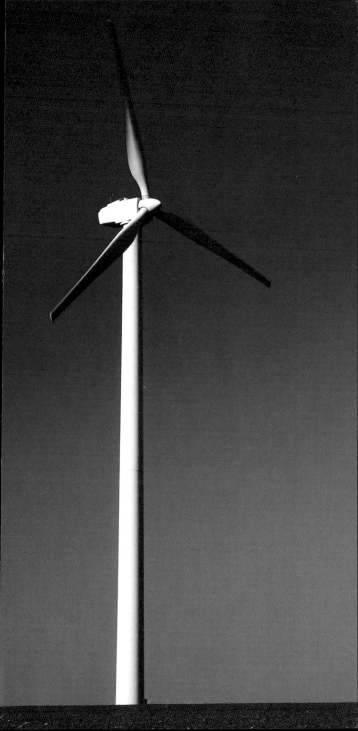

Cognitive behavioural therapy

Cognitive behaviour therapy (or CBT) is used widely in the treatment of IBS. Put simply, CBT is a way of changing how you think (cognitive) and what you do (behaviour). CBT can help to improve your IBS symptoms by breaking them down into manageable parts, working out how they are connected and seeing how they ultimately affect you.

In the UK, CBT is not practised widely so finding a therapist can be difficult. CBT sessions can take place in small groups or on an individual basis. Each session usually lasts about half an hour. Between visits to your therapist you may find it useful to keep a diary to help identify your thought patterns and emotions and how they tie in with your IBS symptoms. The therapist will then help you to work out how to turn any unhelpful thoughts and behaviours into positive ones.

Relaxation therapy

Relaxation is a simple technique that can be easily learnt from audiotapes. It teaches you how to calm your mind by releasing the tension in your body and relaxing your muscles. The idea is that, once your muscles are relaxed, your mind relaxes too. For this reason it can be especially useful in those people for whom stress and anxiety can make their IBS worse.

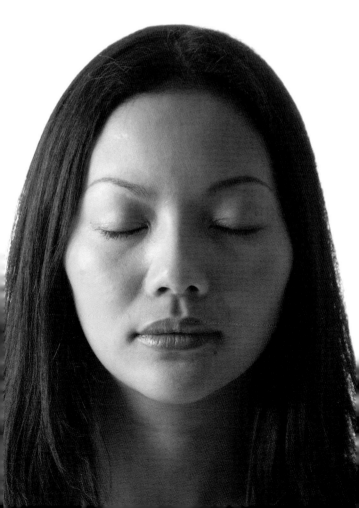

Biofeedback

Biofeedback is about getting a person to understand how their body should be working, and teaching them to recognise when something is going wrong. Biofeedback uses machines to measure and display bodily functions (like heart rate, skin temperature and muscle tension). The patient can then monitor these functions and see how and why they change at different times (i.e. during 'good' and 'bad' IBS days). The idea is that ultimately, by learning to recognise and understand their feelings, the patient will be able to control them.

Biofeedback can make a person more aware of their bowel sensations. Biofeedback recordings can help just about everybody with IBS to recognise when their intestinal tract is about to react abnormally – before they would normally notice symptoms. They can then do something about it before symptoms develop. Biofeedback is usually taught by a qualified physician, nurse or occupational therapist. The key to success is being prepared to practice what you have learnt at home.

Acupuncture

Acupuncture is an ancient Chinese medical treatment that involves the insertion of very fine needles into the body at specific points. There are around 500 acupuncture points all over the body. By mapping 'energy pathways' throughout the body, acupuncture affects the way certain organs, including your bowels, work.

At your first consultation, an acupuncturist will ask you about your symptoms, your medical history and your health in general. They may also feel the quality, rhythm and strength of the pulses on both of your wrists. It is important that you choose an acupuncturist who is suitably qualified. The British Acupuncture Council (*www.acupuncture.org.uk*) will be able to advise you. Because IBS is a chronic condition and persists over long periods of time, you may require regularly scheduled treatments over several months.

Acupuncture comes from the Latin 'acus' (meaning needle) and 'pungere' (meaning prick).

Transcutaneous nerve stimulation (TENS)

TENS is a type of pain relief that involves using small electrical currents to 'block out' the nerves that are transmitting the feelings of pain you associate with IBS. Instead of pain, you will feel more tolerable tingling sensations. Small pads are placed above or to either side of the area that is giving pain, and the results are usually felt straight away. TENS may not work for everyone, however. For people with pacemakers, women in the first 3 months of pregnancy and people who operate heavy machinery, TENS is not appropriate.

Psychotherapy

This is probably what most of us picture when we think of 'therapy'. Psychotherapy usually involves direct personal contact between the therapist and patient. It is a 'talking treatment' and will usually involve the discussion of the often sensitive topics that surround your IBS.

Colonic irrigation

Also known as colonic hydrotherapy, colonic irrigation is a cleansing treatment that is very much in vogue at the moment. The technique involves introducing warm, purified water into the colon via the rectum. The water helps to purge the colon of old waste material and may help to improve muscle contraction and restore the balance of gut microflora. Although many people with IBS say that they benefit from colonic irrigation, no official clinical trials have been conducted to date.

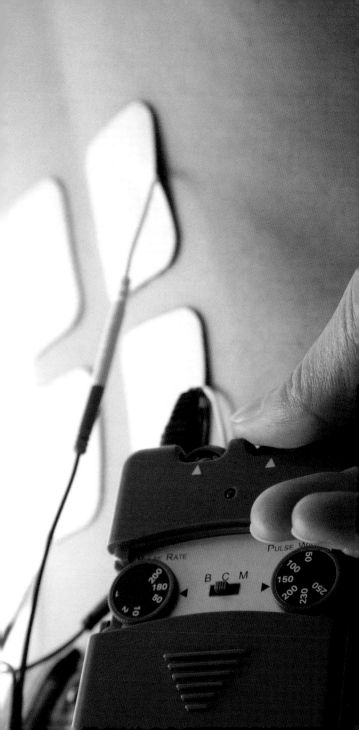

Herbal and dietary supplements for IBS

Herbal and dietary supplements can play an important part in the long-term management of IBS. That said, always proceed with caution when dealing with herbal supplements and use them in strict accordance with their instructions. Claims regarding their effectiveness and safety are generally not reinforced by well-designed clinical trials performed in lots of people (this is in contrast to drugs, which have to go through strict testing procedures before they can be widely used in people).

Always keep your doctor informed of any supplements you are using to control your IBS, in case these interfere with the programme of care that they are recommending.

New European Union directives aiming to offer tighter regulation of these kinds of products are being implemented in the UK, but are not all in force as yet. If you are considering using herbal supplements to control your IBS, always consider the advice of the Medicines Control Agency (MCA).

- Never buy herbal products abroad, from mail order or the internet.
- Only buy a herbal remedy if it states clearly which herbs it contains.
- Make sure you check the dosage of herbs contained in the supplement.
- Stop using herbal remedies if you experience any side-effects.
- Do not exceed the stated dose.
- Do not use if you are pregnant or breast-feeding.
- Use with particular caution in children.

HERBAL AND DIETARY SUPPLEMENTS THAT MAY HELP TO RELIEVE THE SYMPTOMS OF IBS

Probiotics	Restore the balance of gut microflora by introducing 'healthy' bacteria into the body.
Prebiotics	Help the existing gut microflora to work more effectively.
Turmeric	May alleviate the general symptoms of IBS.
Fennel, ginger, cinnamon or camomile tea	May reduce bloating and relieve flatulence.
Evening primrose, borage and fish oils	Can help to calm down the gastrointestinal tract. Evening primrose oil may be particularly effective in women who experience a worsening of pain and bloating during their menstrual period.

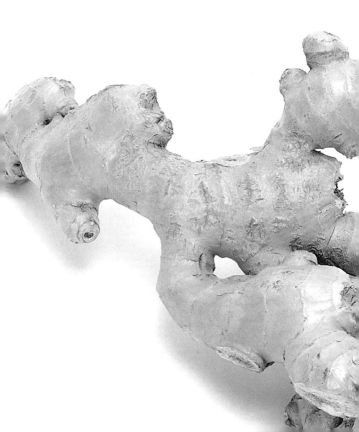

SPECIAL IBS TREATMENT GROUPS

The elderly

Although IBS is a common disorder, it is traditionally considered to largely affect young and middle-aged adults. Of course, many older people will have suffered from IBS for most of their lives and may have had it confirmed at a much earlier age. However, people can sometimes first notice the symptoms of IBS in their later years. Diagnosing IBS in older people is much more difficult than in younger people because it is easier to mistake IBS symptoms for a sign of something else. For this reason, doctors are more likely to order diagnostic tests like barium enemas for their older patients so that they can categorically rule out other diseases.

IBS is treated in much the same way in elderly people, but because they are statistically more likely to suffer from more than one medical complaint, doctors have to take into account whether the IBS medication they are recommending will interfere with other drugs their patient may be taking for other diseases and disorders.

Pregnant women

It is difficult to predict exactly what bearing your pregnancy will have on your IBS. Some women report that their IBS symptoms disappear completely whilst they are pregnant whereas

for others, their IBS becomes worse than ever.
Sometimes, the severity of IBS symptoms may stay
the same whilst the symptoms themselves change
– someone whose IBS is normally diarrhoea-
predominant will suddenly find themselves dealing
with constipation, or *vice versa*.

If your IBS is constipation-predominant
then the chances are it will get worse during
your pregnancy. This may be because of the
physical pressure of the baby on your bowels,
a lack of exercise and changes in the levels of
your hormones.

Ideally, women should take as little
medication as possible during pregnancy. It is
therefore often preferable to use dietary and
lifestyle measures to control IBS rather than
drug treatment.

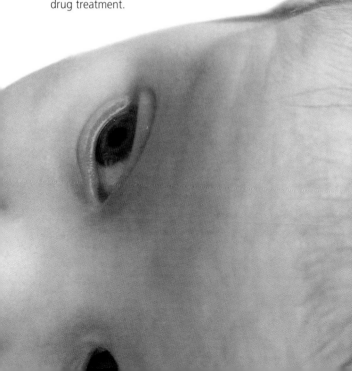

THE LONG AND THE SHORT OF IT

Although IBS is something that will probably affect you on and off for your entire life, if it is properly managed it should not end up dictating what you can and can't do. The various treatments outlined in this section should at least help to improve the symptoms of IBS in the majority of people and, for some, the symptoms will resolve on their own given time. Keep talking to people about your IBS, be they your family, your friends, your doctor or fellow sufferers. The chances are you'll stumble across an IBS solution that works for you.

Currently, IBS medications are not effective for everyone who tries them. This is largely because gaps still remain in our understanding of IBS. Once we work out precisely what causes IBS, we can work out how to treat it more effectively. Given the right research, doctors may one day be able to offer their patients a quick and easy cure for IBS, but until then, people living with the condition should be treated with the respect and compassion they deserve.

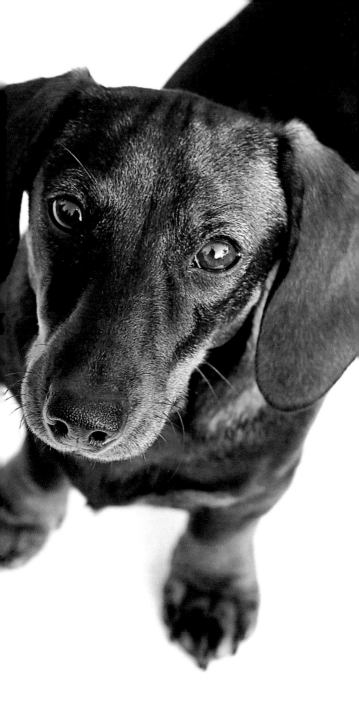

GETTING THE MOST OUT OF YOUR HEALTH SERVICE

When you are first diagnosed with IBS, although it may seem like quite the opposite, try to see your diagnosis as a positive thing. Depending on how bad your symptoms were and how worried you were about them, having IBS confirmed may feel like a tremendous weight has been lifted from your shoulders. Now that you know what's been causing your symptoms, you can work out how best to manage them.

When dealing with IBS, it is important that you find a doctor who will take your symptoms and concerns seriously. Once you've established a good relationship with your GP (or indeed your specialist) they should set out an appropriate management plan for you. Your doctor should:

- sympathise with you and not belittle your symptoms
- reassure you
- explain why you are feeling this way
- set out a sensible personal IBS management plan for you
- help you to take responsibility for your IBS.

Visiting your doctor or any healthcare professional can sometimes be a confusing or daunting prospect. You may find that the consultation flies by and when your doctor asks if you have any questions, your mind goes blank. Writing down a list of questions before the consultation may help you to get the most out of your appointment.

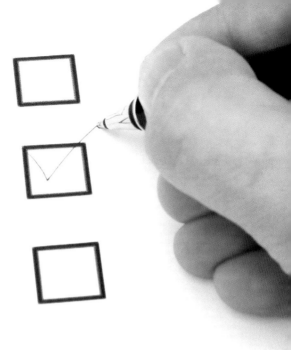

HOW YOU CAN HELP YOUR HEALTH SERVICE TO HELP YOU

■ Don't be afraid to keep going back to your doctor if you don't see any positive changes in your IBS symptoms.

■ Keep a diary of your symptoms, noting down those times and circumstances during which things get especially bad (or good).

■ Stay in regular contact. Report any worsening of symptoms or drug-related side-effects to your doctor immediately.

■ Ask your doctor to explain any advice they give you. Understanding why something should improve your symptoms can really help you get to grips with your IBS.

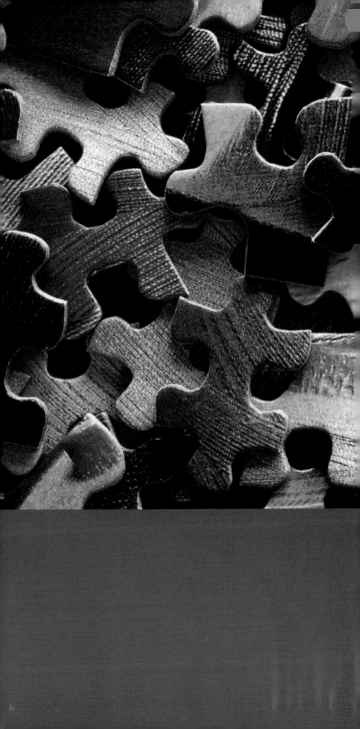

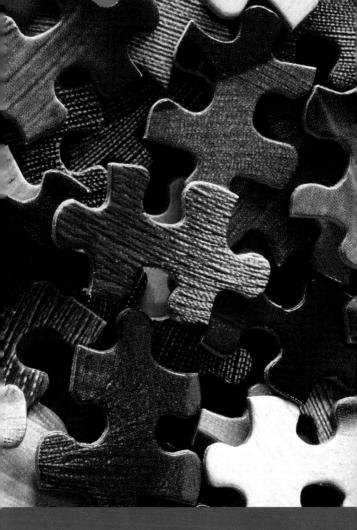

Simple
extras

FURTHER READING

- **_Thyroid disorders (Simple Guide)_**
  CSF Medical Communications Ltd, 2006
  ISBN: 1-905466-09-9, £5.99
  www.bestmedicine.com

USEFUL CONTACTS

- **British Acupuncture Foundation**
  63 Jeddo Road
  London
  W12 9HQ
  Tel: 020 8735 0400
  Email: _info@acupuncture.org.uk_
  Website: _www.acupuncture.org.uk_

- **British Association for Counselling and Psychotherapy**
  BACP House
  35–37 Albert Street
  Rugby
  Warwickshire
  CV21 2SG
  Tel: 0870 4435252
  Email: _bacp@bacp.co.uk_
  Website: _www.bacp.co.uk_

- **British Nutrition Foundation**
  High Holborn House
  52–54 High Holborn
  London
  WC1V 6RQ
  Tel: 020 7404 6504
  Email: _postbox@nutrition.org.uk_
  Website: _www.nutrition.org.uk_

■ **CORE (Digestive Disorders Foundation)**
3 St Andrews Place
London
NW1 4LB
Email: *info@corecharity.org.uk*
Website: *www.digestivedisorders.org.uk*

■ **IBS Network**
Unit 5
53 Mowbray Street
Sheffield
S3 8EN
Helpline: 01142 723253
Email: *info@ibsnetwork.org.uk*
Website: *www.ibsnetwork.org.uk*

■ **NHS Smoking Adviceline**
0800 1690169

■ **Primary Care Society for Gastroenterology**
Gable House
40 High Street
Rickmansworth
Hertfordshire
WD3 1ER
Tel: 01923 712711
Email: *secretariat@pcsg.org.uk*
Website: *www.pcsg.org.uk*

■ **The Hypnotherapy Society**
PO Box 885
Cheltenham
GL53 7WZ
Tel: 0845 6024585
Email: *info@hypnotherapysociety.com*
Website: *www.hypnotherapysociety.com*

YOUR RIGHTS

As a patient, you have a number of important rights. These include the right to the best possible standard of care, the right to information, the right to dignity and respect, the right to confidentiality and underpinning all of these, the right to good health.

Occasionally, you may feel as though your rights have been compromised, or you may be unsure of where you stand when it comes to qualifying for certain treatments or services. In these instances, there are a number of organisations you can turn to for help and advice. Remember that lodging a complaint against your health service should not compromise the quality of care you receive, either now or in the future.

■ **The Patients Association**
The Patients Association (*www.patients-association.com*) is a UK charity which represents patient rights, influences health policy and campaigns for better patient care.
Contact details:
PO Box 935
Harrow
Middlesex
HA1 3YJ
Helpline: 0845 6084455
Email: *mailbox@patients-association.com*

■ **Citizens Advice Bureau**
The Citizens Advice Bureau (*www.nacab.org.uk*) provides free, independent and confidential advice to NHS patients at a number of outreach centres located throughout the country (*www.adviceguide.org.uk*).
Contact details:
Find your local Citizens Advice Bureau using the search tool at *www.citizensadvice.org.uk*.

■ **Patient Advice and Liaison Services (PALS)**

Set up by the Department of Health (*www.dh.gov.uk*), PALS provide information, support and confidential advice to patients, families and their carers.

Contact details:

Phone your local hospital, clinic, GP surgery or health centre and ask for details of the PALS, or call NHS Direct on 0845 46 47.

■ **The Independent Complaints Advocacy Service (ICAS)**

ICAS is an independent service that can help you bring about formal complaints against your NHS practitioner. ICAS provides support, help, advice and advocacy from experienced advisors and caseworkers.

Contact details:

ICAS Central Team

Myddelton House

115–123 Pentonville Road

London N1 9LZ

Email: *icascentralteam@citizensadvice.org.uk*

Or contact your local ICAS office direct.

Accessing your medical records

You have a legal right to see all your health records under the Data Protection Act of 1998. You can usually make an informal request to your doctor and you should be given access within 40 days. Note that you may have to pay a small fee for the privilege.

You can be denied access to your records if your doctor believes that the information contained within them could cause serious harm to you or another person. If you are applying for access on behalf of someone else, then you will not be granted access to information which the patient gave to his or her doctor on the understanding that it would remain confidential.

PERSONAL RECORD:

My Simple Guide

This Simple Guide belongs to:

Name:

Address:

Tel:

Email:

In case of emergency please contact:

Name:

Address:

Tel:

Email:

My Healthcare Team

GP surgery address and telephone number

Name: _____

Address: _____

_____

_____

Tel: _____

I am registered with Dr _____

_____

My dietitian _____

My pharmacist _____

My therapist _____

Other members of my healthcare team

_____

_____

_____

FOOD DIARY

Keeping a record of the foods you eat and how they tie-in with your IBS symptoms can help you to take control of your IBS.

Date:

Time	Description of food eaten	Symptoms experienced
Breakfast		
Mid-morning		
Lunch		
Mid-afternoon		

Date:

Time	Description of food eaten	Symptoms experienced
Evening meal		
Rest of evening		
Units of alcohol		
Forgotten snacks		

NOTES

NOTES

NOTES

NOTES

NOTES

SIMPLE GUIDE QUESTIONNAIRE

Dear reader,

We would love to know what you thought of this
Simple Guide. Please take a few moments to fill out this
short questionnaire and return it to us at the FREEPOST
address below.

CSF Medical Communications Ltd
FREEPOST NAT5703
Witney
OX29 8BR

SO WHAT DID YOU THINK?

Which Simple Guide have you just read?

_____

Where did you buy it (store/town)?

_____

Who did you buy it for?
☐ Myself   ☐ Friend   ☐ Relative
☐ Patient   ☐ Other

Where did you hear about the Simple Guides?
☐ They were recommended to me   ☐ Internet
☐ Stumbled across them   ☐ Other

Did it meet with your expectations?
☐ Exceeded   ☐ Met all
☐ Met most   ☐ Fell below

Was there anything you particularly liked?

_____

_____

_____

Was there anything we could have improved?

_____

_____

_____

WHO ARE YOU?

Name: _____

Address: _____

_____

_____

Tel: _____

Email: _____

How old are you?

☐ Under 25   ☐ 25–34   ☐ 35–44
☐ 45–54   ☐ 55–64   ☐ 65+

Are you...   ☐ Male   ☐ Female

Do you suffer from a long-term medical condition? If so, please specify.

_____

WHAT NEXT?

What other topics would you like to see covered in future Simple Guides?

Thanks,
  the Simple Guides team